Advance Praise for *Th*

"Discover the power of ho
gods, modern cure, and l
fascinating book."

> —Dr. Ava Cadell, author and founder of
> Loveology University

"I'm amazed at all the great health benefits that can be had from honey. I have fresh organic bee pollen in my freezer and local organic honey on my table. Thanks, Cal, for all your good work informing people about honey."

> —Sherry Henderson, Editor/Publisher,
> *Oracle 20/20 Magazine*

"Cal Orey has done a wonderful job of thoroughly explaining the great value of honey. *The Healing Powers of Honey* is an easy-to-read book that's an invaluable addition to anyone's library. It's full of practical tips and applications for medical conditions that everyone should know about."

> —Allan Magaziner, D.O.
> Magaziner Center for Wellness
> Cherry Hill, New Jersey

"An original book using the queen honey bee and human metaphors in anecdotes is charming and witty. Pairing olive oil and honey in cooking and baking is healthful. *The Healing Powers of Honey* is a masterpiece."

> —Gemma Sanita Sciabica, author of the
> *Cooking with California Olive Oil* series

"Cal Orey scores again with *The Healing Powers of Honey,* a continuation of her widely praised *Healing Powers* series. Orey's honey book is well researched in a manner that makes it both entertaining and informative. This book will

make you look at honey in a new way—as a bona fide health food as well as a gastronomic treat."
—Joe Traynor, agriculturist-author of
Honey: The Gourmet Medicine

"Not everyone can be a beekeeper, but Cal Orey shares the secrets that honey bees and their keepers have always known. Honey is good for body and soul."
—Kim Flottum, editor of *Bee Culture* magazine and author of *The Backyard Beekeeper, The Honey Handbook,* and *Better Beekeeping*

Books by Cal Orey

The Healing Powers of Vinegar
The Healing Powers of Olive Oil
The Healing Powers of Chocolate

Published by Kensington Publishing Corporation

The Healing Powers of

HONEY

A Complete Guide to Nature's Remarkable Nectar

CAL OREY

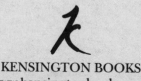

KENSINGTON BOOKS
www.kensingtonbooks.com

Permission to reproduce The Mediterranean Diet Pyramid and Common Foods and Flavors of the Mediterranean Diet Pyramid © 2009, granted by Oldways Preservation & Exchange Trust, www.oldwayspt.org

KENSINGTON BOOKS are published by

Kensington Publishing Corp.
119 West 40th Street
New York, NY 10018

Copyright © 2011 by Cal Orey

All Kensington titles, imprints, and distributed lines are available at special quantity discounts for bulk purchases for sales promotion, premiums, fund-raising, educational, or institutional use. Special book excerpts or customized printings can also be created to fit specific needs. For details, write or phone the office of the Kensington Special Sales Manager: Attn. Special Sales Department. Kensington Publishing Corp., 119 West 40th Street, New York, NY 10018. Phone: 1-800-221-2647.

Kensington and the K logo Reg. U.S. Pat & TM Off.

ISBN-13: 978-1-4967-1254-7
ISBN-10: 1-4967-1254-4
First Kensington Trade Edition: October 2011
First Kensington Mass Market Edition: March 2018

eISBN-13: 978-0-7582-7455-7
eISBN-10: 0-7582-7455-6
First Kensington Electronic Edition: March 2018

10 9 8 7 6 5

Printed in the United States of America

Warning: To avoid infant botulism, do not feed honey to a baby who is younger than one year.

This book is dedicated to the honey bees—especially the persevering workers and queens—whom I feel are my kindred spirits. I feel a strong and moving bond to this small but remarkable hardworking creature with big efforts—nature's greatest gift.

CONTENTS

Foreword

A "sweet treat" that is good for you? What sugar can be eaten without guilt and bring you health benefits? What delectable substance comes in as many flavors as fine wine? The answers to these questions all point to one natural food—pure, natural honey!

This delicious treat is what some call nature's sweetener. But honey is so much more. It is a superfood that from ancient times has been known for its healthful and nutritional properties. It is a food that can be eaten in moderation without guilt. Cal Orey shows you why honey should be consumed daily for your health. So if you already love honey, or perhaps have never eaten it, or would love to have a good reason to love it, this book is a must-read.

HONEY HIGHLIGHTS

Bridging history and contemporary science, *The Healing Powers of Honey* presents a reader-friendly gem to explain the therapeutic and health benefits of honey. These amazing benefits include a lowered risk for heart disease, high blood pressure, diabetes, and obesity, an enhanced immune system function, and a longer, healthier life. Simply put, honey has been touted for its concentrated energy, as it is loaded with flavonoids and dozens of other active ingredients that are needed by the body.

For centuries, mankind has survived because of the medicinal benefits of nature's finest foods that prevent disease or even heal and cure. *The Healing Powers of Honey* resolves any conflict between folklore and traditional medicine concerning honey by bridging time with facts drawn from a variety of sources. The proof is in the honey—and Cal Orey shows it chapter by chapter in this revolutionary book.

A POUND OF SWEET RESEARCH

It has been my privilege as the co-chairman of the Committee for the Promotion of Honey and Health, Inc., for the past several years to research and write about the health benefits of honey. Thanks to my brother-in-law, a commercial beekeeper in Kansas, I have moved from skeptic to believer. Along with a pharmacist from Edinburgh, Scotland, we have scoured the world's literature for information relating to healing honey. Though much of the medical and scientific information about honey comes from smaller observational studies completed outside the United States, it is no less valid than results from large research projects accomplished in our backyard under well-controlled studies.

A good example is found in discovering the effects of honey on human metabolism. Honey regulates and stabilizes blood sugar. That statement on the surface seems as counterintuitive as eating bacon to control one's cholesterol. Yet multiple observations have indicated that the consumption of honey on a regular basis actually lowers blood-sugar levels and helps prevent swings in blood sugar throughout the day and during sleep and exercise.

The fact that honey, a combination of two simple sugars—both fructose and glucose—is able to regulate and control blood sugar is confirmed by understanding basic human physiology. Both sugars, found in honey in a near equal ratio, are required for the formation of most of the glycogen made and stored in the liver. It is this action following eating honey that is responsible for many of honey's miraculous health benefits in *The Healing Powers of Honey*.

Other health benefits from honey, from ancient folk medicine to modern miracle, include aiding in treatment of ailments including digestion, insomnia, coughs, and respiratory diseases, helping improve skin conditions, enhancing sport performance, and much more.

Another powerful and therapeutic benefit of honey comes not from its consumption but in its external use. Study after study has shown that honey shows powerful antimicrobial properties. Some honey varietals, such as manuka honey, produced from nectar from the manuka plant in New Zealand and Australia, have been found to be very effective in treating wounds, although all types of honeys are helpful.

Human-Friendly Honey Varietals

While manuka honey is touted for its powers around the globe, other honey varietals, such as buckwheat honey, have been found to contain higher levels of antioxidants. Buckwheat honey, used in a cough suppressant study at Penn State University Medical School, was found to be superior to the most common over-the-counter cough suppressant available.

The question is frequently asked of me, "What kind of honey is the best?" The answer really depends on one's taste. All honey is good as well as good for you. Honey is like wine. There are as many varietals of honey as there are floral and nectar sources. "Try several" is the best advice in choosing honey for your family. Select honey that is from identifiable floral sources and choose the ones that please your palate.

Finally, *The Healing Powers of Honey* has accomplished what no promotional campaign can or would do. The facts about honey and its powerful healthful and healing benefits are now mainstream, no longer relegated to folklore. All of us can celebrate the historic and healthful benefits of the wonder natural food given to us by the Creator as we experience the healing powers of honey for ourselves—with gratitude to Cal for her delightful and informative work.

—Ronald E. Fessenden, M.D., M.P.H.,
co-author of *The Honey Revolution:
Restoring the Health of Future Generations*

Preface

On a cold winter day, I was sipping a cup of chamomile tea laced with orange blossom honey. Nature's finest sweetener with my beverage of choice comforted me. After all, I wasn't working on a book like an author should be to feel in the comfort zone. An unexpected e-mail from my book editor surprised me. He asked me if I was interested in writing another *Healing Powers* book. The words "garlic" and "fruit juices" were put on the table—but I had my own superfood choice in mind.

During the creation of *The Healing Powers of Chocolate*, I noticed that honey, like chocolate, was noted in the Mediterranean diet. It was the first sign that writing a book on another food of the gods was in the stars for me. And that five-letter word—"h-o-n-e-y"—stuck in my mind like a honey bee on a sunflower. Later, when I was a guest on national radio programs to talk about the virtues of chocolate a few hosts asked me the question "What's the topic of your next book?" Without hesitation I darted, "Honey." What else could follow the class act of decadent chocolate, right? So I put the idea on the back burner.

The topic of honey came back to me and I'm glad it

did. When I was faced with a new book proposition and providing another healing food, it was a no-brainer. I wrote a message stating: "I was waiting for this day to happen. Honey!" and e-mailed it to my editor, Richard Ember. One week later, the night before honey went to the editors' meeting, I tuned into TV and the film *Fried Green Tomatoes* greeted me. The protagonist (Jessica Tandy) plays an interesting character and a "bee charmer"—young and old. To me, it was another cue that my proposed topic was going to be a thumbs-up. Also, that night the America Online stationery available to users, like me, offered a picture of a bee, flower, and honeycomb background with the word "honey" in the bottom right-hand corner. It was another message. And the next day, Saint Patrick's Day, with a bit of luck of the Irish, it was confirmed. I was assigned the new book project—*The Healing Powers of Honey*. It was meant to be.

By being a California native (a popular home of bee-keepers who rely on both sales of honey and the honey bee for pollination of our fruits, vegetables, and nuts) I was given the ticket to enter the land of honey.

Like vinegar, olive oil, and chocolate, honey is derived from nature. The four books tout health benefits from these disease-fighting, antioxidant-rich foods, from ancient folk medicine to modern miracles.

So, like a worker bee, I began my quest. I delved into my work. It was my goal this time around to find out the past and present gifts of honey. The exciting part of my journey is that I discovered that the hardworking, goal-oriented honey bee plays an integral part in our ecosystem and survival of mankind.

Once again, I find myself sitting in my study writing a *Healing Powers* book. This time around, I'm drinking tea infused with tupelo honey, savoring a honey chocolate truffle, and feeling the softness of my fingers from honey soap as I work on the keyboard. Oh, and honey-apple muffins are baking in the oven. In *The Healing Powers of Honey* I'll show you how and why this natural "nectar of the gods" will transcend your awareness of the sacred honey bee and its remarkable gift to you.

Acknowledgments

Like a forager honey bee, during the 1970s I hitchhiked across America in search of Shangri-la and a home. Today, in the 21st century as a hardworking author I would like to express my heartfelt thanks to the contributions of the National Honey Board, The Honey Association, my publisher at Kensington, and my editor, Richard Ember, who has guided me through the *Healing Powers* series.

Thanks also go to the honey companies, beekeepers, scientists, and health researchers in the United States and around the globe that helped me understand how important the sacred honey bee is to mankind.

PART 1

A TIME FOR HONEY

The Power of Honey

*Honey comes out of the air . . . At early
dawn the leaves, of trees are found bedewed
with honey . . . It is always of the best
quality when it is stored in the best flowers.*
—Pliny (A.D. 23–79)[1]

As a child, in my dreams I lived in a cottage with my father, a dedicated beekeeper, and mom, who did all cooking, canning, and baking with honey. In our garden I'd watch my father experiment with hives and establish an apiary on 10 acres. He shipped Italian queen bees across the United States and around the world. But my home was normal, because in reality I grew up in a middle-class suburb of south San Jose, California, a place once touted for its nectar sources—a honey bee's dreamworld.

My first encounter with honey was when I was five years old. In kindergarten I remember drawing a giant honey bee on a wildflower. (It didn't hold a beeswax candle to beekeeper Prince Cesi's microscopic drawing of the insect.) After art time, Mrs. Berry dished out graham crackers (sweetened with honey and developed by Sylvester Graham in 1829), milk cartons, and Mr. Bee-Good notes (little square papers with special kudos to three good students once a week). When I wasn't one of the chosen few, my mind wandered; *What would life be like as a bee?* My imagination soared with images of me morphing into an insect and flying from flower to flower to fill up on sweet nectar.

That was decades ago, and today I can look back at my life experiences and see how the honey bee and honey played a role in my real world. I wasn't raised by a beekeeper and his wife, nor as a kid did I put on a bee veil and visit bees. But I got a taste of honey and its healing powers throughout the years of growing up and traveling like a wayward bee.

Today, I sit here in my hive-like wood-paneled study and I feel the spirit of the honey bee as I work on *The Healing Powers of Honey*. My file cabinet behind me is full of material on everything from honeycomb to honey candies. In my kitchen pantry, honeys—dozens of healthful dark and light varieties—sit. The best part is, I have discovered the healing magic of honey, and a world I've called Honeyland that I want to share with you.

HONEY 101: NATURE'S GIFT

Honey, one of the oldest sweeteners, comes from flower nectar that has been consumed by the honey bee (*Apis mellifera*), which was originally found in Europe. (The Entomological Society of America uses two words, "honey bee," and the British use one word, "honeybee.") Known as "nectar of the gods," as far back as

5,000 years ago it was used for medicinal purposes, in cooking and as a preservative, as a medicinal agent, in cosmetics, and in soaps, and even the beeswax has been used for candles.

> *Honey: a sweet viscid material elaborated out of the nectar of flowers in the honey sac of various bees.*
> —Merriam-Webster's Collegiate Dictionary, 11th edition

The Honey Makers: So, how exactly do honey bees make honey, anyhow? They diligently collect nectar from flowers and other plants and carry it to the hive. It's those honey bees that are responsible for transforming the floral nectar that they gather into honey by adding enzymes to the nectar and reducing moisture.

The honey bee full of nectar comes back to the hive and goes to work. Honey is stored in hexagonal chambers. The honeycomb structure of the hive also has rooms for the queen bee to lay her eggs. Before honey is available to put in your tea or on top of a muffin, the honey-covered walls of the hive are removed and placed in a spinner. Rotated fast, the spinner separates the liquid from the comb.

Once extracted straight from the hive, honey is a combination of fructose, glucose, and water. This sweet gift also contains other sugars, enzymes, minerals, vitamins, amino acids, and, most important, many types of honeys boast antioxidants—the good-for-you compounds that can help keep your body inside and outside healthy and boost your life span.

. . . And Key Pollinators: Beekeepers know that honey bees provide another service; as second-shift workers they pollinate one-third of the food we eat. As a bee travels in search of nectar, it brushes against pollen-bearing parts of a flower and picks up pollen. When the honey bee goes to another flower for more food, some of the pollen from the first flower sticks to the second flower—and the flower is pollinated.

The honey bee pollinates more than 90 crops, including apples, blueberries, citrus fruit, and nuts—approximately four-fifths of the fresh fruits and vegetables we eat. Indeed, hardworking honey bee colonies (50,000 to 60,000 bees per hive, including workers, drones, and one queen) who work double duty (like hardworking humans) are man's best friends because they are vital to our planet.

"Honey bees are woven into our food chain. Without honey bees the whole food chain would be diminished in diversity and quantity for us," explains Hidden Valley Honey's beekeeper Chris Foster of Reno, Nevada, who lives 50 miles away from me—and showed me his colonies in action and their products, from buzzing bees to fresh honey in jars.

HONEY FORMS TO TASTE

Like more than 50 percent of American households, you may have liquid honey in your kitchen cupboard, but there are a variety of forms of honey available for both your health and enjoyment, too.

Form	Description of Honey	Taste and Texture
Comb Honey	Attached to the comb from the hive	Fresh bits of wax, chewy
Crystallized	Liquid honey that has crystallized due to sugar content of the honey having separated from the liquid	Not a preferred texture
Cut Comb or Liquid Honey	Contains chunks of honeycomb	Combination of of liquid and wax, chewy and syrupy
Liquid Honey	The most popular type of honey, clear without crystals, often used in baking or drizzled on food	Syrupy
Whipped or Creamed Honey	Crystallized during manufacturing, preferred in many countries	Thick, spreadable, creamy

(*Source:* National Honey Board.)

FROM SWEET NECTAR TO SUPER HONEY

Not only are there different forms of honey to eat, but there are a variety of honeys, touted by people—from foodies to health nuts—as one of Mother Nature's superfoods (like antioxidant-rich chocolates and olive oils). And now healing honeys in a variety of flavors are making the news around the world and are popular in restaurants, beauty spas, and our homes.

Honey is not just a liquid sweetener that you put in your tea or on your toast. It's an ancient medicine that has been used to treat heart disease, respiratory ailments, skin ulcers, wounds, stomach problems, insomnia, and even "superbugs." Honey is also known to help curb sweet cravings and boost energy, which can help stave off type 2 diabetes, unwanted pounds, and body fat.

Top scientists, nutritionists, and medical doctors know stacks and stacks of research show some honeys contain the same disease-fighting antioxidant compounds that are found in fruits and vegetables, which fight heart disease, cancers, diabetes, and obesity—four problems in the United States and around the world.

SuperFoods HealthStyle co-author Steven G. Pratt, M.D., world-renowned authority on nutrition, points out that certain superfoods keep you healthy and stave off diseases: "Perhaps honey's most important health-promoting benefit is its antioxidant ability. We know that daily consumption of honey raises blood levels of protective antioxidants."[2]

Jonny Bowden, Ph.D., author of *The 150 Healthiest Foods on Earth: The Surprising, Unbiased Truth About What You Should Eat and Why,* also praises raw, unfiltered honey: "Honey is pure alchemy. And it's precious stuff." It's common consensus among beekeepers that the real, raw, unprocessed, unheated, unfiltered kind of honey that you get you get straight from the hive—honeycomb—is the real deal with good-for-you antioxidants. Think pure apple cider vinegar, unadulterated olive oil, and quality dark cocoa: raw honey, like these antioxidant-rich superfoods, is the healthy stuff.[3]

Most medical doctors and nutritionists I spoke with during my trek through Honeyland agreed that while honey is a sugar, it does contain disease-fighting antioxidants and other health virtues that make it the standout sweetener of choice.

Health-Boosting Nutrients in Honey

Medical researchers around the world continue to find new health-promoting nutrients in honeys. Most important, like red wine, green tea, and certain fruits and vegetables, honey contains antioxidants—disease-fighting enzymes that protect your body by trapping free-radical molecules. (Imagine video game–like bright yellow Pac-Man heads, with mouths that open and close like a shark, chasing big bad bugs and gobbling them up before any damage occurs to a human body.)

Research also shows that eating antioxidant-rich superfoods— like honey—may lower the risk of developing diseases and even stall the aging process. Researchers continue to find new health-promoting nutrients in certain superfoods, and here are some of the super ones in honey that you should know about:

Alpha-tocopherol: an essential antioxidant, known as vitamin E.

Enzymes: chemical substances your body produces to help boast chemical reactions in your body.

Flavanols and Flavonols: a group of plant compounds (from flavonoids, a large group of phytonutrients) found in honey that have shown antioxidant effects that may help lower the risk of developing heart disease, some forms of cancer, and diabetes. Both flavanols and flavonols can be found in honey.

Oligosaccharides: aids to heart health, by lowering blood pressure and cholesterol, and regularity, by boosting good bacteria in the colon.

Peptides: molecules made up of two or more linked amino acids that may help lower risk of heart disease, too, as well as enhance the immune system and digestion.

Polyphenols: natural compounds that act as powerful antioxidants to protect your body by trapping the free-radical molecules and getting rid of them before damage occurs.

Salicylates: naturally produced acid that acts as a protective compound against stress and disease.

(Sources: The *Healing Powers* series, *Super-Foods HealthStyle*, and *The 150 Healthiest Foods on Earth*.)

HONEY VARIETALS

Honey is made from a wide variety of flowers, trees, and other plants. There are hundreds of varieties found around the world. It's the darkest honeys that are the ones to write home about, because these are the super-stars with medicinal value that deserve kudos in the human world.

The following 10 flavors of honeys—some of the top antioxidant-rich and medicinal ones—are listed alpha-betically. These honeys are sitting side by side in jars (hex shaped to bear shaped) in my pantry. One by one, I encountered each flavor, and today I use each one of them for its unique healing benefits. I dish out more details for you about the honey varietals in my up close and personal experiences with you in chapter 7.

THE HEALING HONEY PARADE

Type	Characteristics	Nectar Source
Acacia	Light, white-yellowish; medicinal	Black locust tree
Blueberry	Golden in color; rich in antioxidants	A flowering shrub with pale flowers
Buckwheat	Dark and rich; high in antioxidants	Annual herb
Goldenrod	Amber, golden; medicinal	A perennial with branches of golden flowers

Hawaiian Christmas Berry	Rich golden; high in antioxidants	Christmas berry bush
Manuka	Dark amber-orange; medicinal	Manuka bush
Sidr	Superdark amber; medicinal	Ancient sidr tree
Raspberry	Pale yellow; medicinal	American red raspberry shrub
Sunflower	Yellow; medicinal	An annual herb with daisy-like flowers
Wildflower	Light golden; medicinal	Variety of wild-flowers

HEALING PRODUCTS FROM THE HIVE

Honey is healing, but its bee products straight from the hive also have healing powers, the practice of which is known as "apitherapy." While honey types and forms do come with health perks, four by-products straight from the hive are also creating a buzz. I learned that these gifts for both bees and mankind can be and are used for health and healing and in the home. Thanks to the human honey producers, my pantry is chock-full of not only honey varietals, but also other bee foods that are making news around the globe.

Pollen: A protein-rich, powder-like substance. Honey bees gather pollen as food for themselves and their young. Bee pollen is packed with vitamins, minerals, enzymes, and amino acids. It has more amino acids and vitamins that any other amino acid–containing product, like beef, eggs, or cheese, claim nutritionists. People in the honey world recommend starting slowly and building up to 1 to 2 teaspoons of pollen each day. Some people will use pollen in cereal, smoothies, and yogurt, and a few chocolatiers include it in their chocolates. Find pollen at health-food stores and specialty honey shops.

Propolis: A sticky, dark-colored, waxy sap collected by honey bees from the buds of trees. Used by honey bees to close up cracks. People use it as a disinfectant as well as to treat a number of health ailments, including an oncoming cold. It is found in different forms, including chews, a spray, tincture, raw chunks, and capsules. Chews and propolis are available at health-food stores and honey specialty shops. When I opened a jar of bee propolis raw honey product from Dutchman's Gold Inc. and Annie's Apitherapy I was greeted with a thin layer of dark stuff on top. At first, I thought, *A bee gift of sorts.* I assumed it was propolis but wanted to know before I took a nibble. The mystery black layer was bee propolis. (Nutritional consultant Angela Ysseldyk, www.beepollenbuzz.com, recommends mixing it in. Simply heat the honey [do not microwave it] by placing the jar in a pot on the stove until it begins to melt. Do this slowly and be careful not to overheat and accidentally pasteurize your honey.)

Royal Jelly: A creamy liquid made and secreted by nurse bees to feed the queen. This is a nutrient-rich natural jelly with proteins, amino acids, fatty acids, minerals, sugars, and vitamins. It's touted as a skin product and dietary supplement. Honey lovers and health enthusiasts believe it has many health benefits. I'm told some folks (not me yet) can handle eating royal jelly solo; others (humans, not bees) will mix it with honey to make it easier to swallow. Royal jelly is available fresh in little jars, like honey types, and capsules. (Check out chapter 5: "Honey, You're Amazing!" and chapter 11: "Home Remedies from Your Kitchen" to find its potential healing powers.)

Beeswax: The wax that is processed from the glands of the female honey bee's abdomen. Sure, this isn't for eating, but it is molded to make honeycomb. It can be used for all-natural cosmetics, candles, and furniture polish. (Refer to chapter 12: "Honeymania: Honey for the Household" to find out about these honey products for you and your home.)

10 Honey Buzz-worthy Bits

Since the honey bee and mankind are connected because of our food chain, it makes sense to dish out a spoonful of honey trivia to show you just how the honey bee is an un-bee-lievable man's best friend. Take a look at these 10 factoids that'll get you thinking about the amazing small creature and what it can do.

It takes about 2 million flowers for honey bees to tap to make one pound of honey.

1. The average honey worker bee makes a mere $\frac{1}{12}$ teaspoon of honey in her lifetime.
2. Utah is known as the Beehive State.
3. Honey bees communicate by dancing. The waggle dance alerts other bees to where the nectar and pollen are.
4. A honey bee must tap about 2 million flowers to make 1 pound of honey.

5. On average, each person in the United States consumes about 1.31 pounds of honey each year.
6. The U.S. Department of Agriculture estimates that there are approximately 3 million honey-producing colonies in the United States.
7. It would take about 2 tablespoons of honey to fuel a bee's flight around the world.
8. A worker bee visits about 50 to 100 flowers during each trip.
9. A honey bee flies about 15 miles per hour.
10. A hive of bees flies more than 55,000 miles to bring you one pound of honey.

(*Source:* National Honey Board.)

As you can see, the remarkable honey bee flies the extra mile so it can produce honey—a superfood (a food that has super health benefits) for people, like you and me—that can be enjoyed solo or in a cup of tea or both ways. Here is a perfect recipe to whip up and savor with a cup of tea and honey as you fly away with me on a journey into Honeyland.

Honey Tea Bread

❖ ❖ ❖

8 ounces raisins
3 ounces set honey
½ pint freshly made strong tea
2 large eggs, lightly beaten

10 ounces whole-wheat flour
½ teaspoon ground spice
1 tablespoon baking powder

Place the raisins in a bowl. Stir the honey into the tea and pour this over raisins. Leave to soak for 2 hours. Stir the eggs into the raisin mixture.

Preheat oven to 350°F. Mix the flour with the spice and baking powder, then mix these dry ingredients into the raisin mixture. Transfer to a greased 2-pound loaf tin and bake for about 1 hour 10 minutes.

Cook on a wire rack and serve sliced and buttered. Makes one 2-pound loaf.

(*Courtesy:* The Honey Association.)

Un-bee-lievable Healing Hints to Catch

Research, especially in the past decade, shows that quality dark honeys, which are derived from a variety of flowers, trees, and other plants, produce the nectar for the honey around the globe—and may help you to:

✓ lower your risk of heart disease.
✓ enhance your immune system.

✓ stave off diabetes.
✓ treat respiratory diseases.
✓ heal wounds.
✓ slow the aging process.
✓ add years to your life.

In this book, I will show you how using honey (paired with other superfoods) is one of the best things you can do for yourself—and your health. But note, many people will not want to reap the benefits of honey by indulging in the dark stuff by teaspoons (like dark chocolate, it's an acquired taste). But you can get your daily honey dose from a flavorful cup of tea and honey and in cooking and baking. I've included dozens of recipes to pamper your palate and to help heal your body, mind, and spirit. And versatile honey in foods, cosmetics, soaps, and lotions, medicinal dressings, candles, and furniture polish can do so much more for both the inside and outside of your body and your household.

But first, let's go way, way back into the past. Take a honey bee's–eye view of why and how honey is one of the ancient world's first—and most remarkable—natural medicines.

An Ancient Essential Elixir

*The secret of my health is applying honey
inside and oil outside.*
—Democritus, contemporary of
Hippocrates[1]

My second encounter with honey was when I was a budding tomboy who favored insects and furry creatures,
big and small, rather than toys and dolls. My kindergarten fantasy of having a backyard with flowers, plants,
trees, and weeds with butterflies and honey bees was no
longer a dream. My dad landscaped both our front and
backyard—complete with a large hour glass–shaped
patio. In the spring and summer the backyard was my
refuge. I was mesmerized by the long row of tall bright
red bottlebrush plants—an attraction to active honey
bees. Listening to the sound of daily buzzing was like
watching *The Sound of Music*—an escape from the everyday world.

Not only did the sound and sight of bees in our yard captivate me, but on summer nights honey-glazed chicken sizzling on the barbeque pit was an attraction, too. The scent of a fresh-baked apple pie sweetened with clover honey—cooling on the kitchen counter—wasn't to be ignored, either. After dinner, I'd take a dip in the next-door neighbor's swimming pool. It may not have been Greece, but it was home. My dad sold insurance, not bees or honey. But honey bees in the suburbs were part of my life, as they were noticed in other people's worlds in the 20th century and long ago.

Back in the days of the ancient past, benefits of honey used for medicinal purposes varied from physical stamina to mental well-being. The versatile healing powers of honey were put to work by Egyptian physicians as far as 5,000 years ago, and its medical uses have also been noted in the Old World from traditional Chinese medicine to Indian Ayurveda.[2]

HOLY HONEY HISTORY TIDBITS

Honey is mentioned countless times in the Bible. The phrase "milk and honey" was used at least 21 different places to describe the fertility and prosperity of the Promised Land, in contrast to the desert, which did not flow with water, milk, or honey.

Honey is one of the Bible's good-for-you healing foods. Here are some interesting biblical references to honey—and what they may mean. These were gleaned from a variety of sources, all leading to the Bible:

Honey as in the Land of Milk and Honey

- "Go up to the land flowing with milk and honey. But I will not go with you, because you are a stiff-necked people and I might destroy you" (Exodus 33:3, New International Version).

- "If the LORD is pleased with us, he will lead us into that land, a land flowing with milk and honey, and will give it to us" (Numbers 14:8).

Honey, a Healing Gift

Not only will you find passages of the Holy Bible with references to the Promised Land, but in Genesis 43:11 Jacob sends honey as a gift to Joseph, the governor of Egypt. And in Kings 14:3 Jeroboam requests his spouse to give the gift of honey to the prophet Ahijah, with promise of its healing powers for their son who was allegedly blind.[3]

Honey, the Symbol of Good Health

- "Now the men of Israel were in distress that day, because Saul had bound the people under an oath, saying, Cursed be any man who eats food before evening comes, before I have avenged myself on my enemies! So none of the troops tasted food. The entire army entered the woods, and there was honey on the ground. When they went into the woods, they saw honey oozing out, yet no one put his hand to his mouth, because they feared the oath. But Jonathan had not heard that his father had bound the people with the oath, so he reaches out the end of the staff that was in his hand and dipped it into the honeycomb. He raised his hand to his mouth, and his eyes brightened" (1 Samuel 14:24–27).

Honey, the Ultimate Food

- "Butter and honey shall he eat" (Isaiah 7:15).
- "The people of Israel called the bread manna. It

was white like coriander seed and tasted like wafers made with honey" (Exodus 16:31).

- "The day Christ rose from the dead and appeared before His Disciples, He asked for food. They gave him broiled fish and a honeycomb" (Luke 24:42).
- "My son, eat honey because it is good, and the honeycomb which is sweet to your taste" (Proverbs 24:13).

With all of this being put on today's kitchen table how can you go wrong by adding a little honey in your diet? Honey is praised by people during the ups and downs of biblical times, but the golden nectar doesn't end there. . . .

ODE TO THE SWEET GIFT OF HONEY

Not only is golden honey found in the Old Testament, but it's noted in Greek mythology, too. Remember, Zeus, the legendary son of Cronos, in Greece? Zeus was an almighty god of the sky and king of the gods. Enter Melissa—the meaning is "honey bee"—who nurtured Zeus during the time he was estranged from his father. Melissa fed Zeus honey that she borrowed from beehives. This good feat, in turn, ended up in an evil punishment for the caring woman. Cronos transformed her into a worm. The end result: Zeus was thankful for Melissa's help with the golden nectar and like a good warlock he turned her into a queen bee.[4]

Honey is also known as the nectar of Aphrodite—the Greek goddess of love and beauty. As mythology and folklore enthusiasts tell it, she allegedly pacified Cerberus, the three-headed dog, with a sweet honey cake and paid Charon to take her to Hades. En route, she saw hands reaching out of the water. A voice told her to toss a honey cake to them. She tossed the cake out to the hands and gave one to Cerberus. The sweet gift of honey got the goddess to where she wanted to be.

THE EGYPTIAN SEED OF HONEY . . .

While myths and legends are mind-boggling, inscriptions on Sumerian tables are more believable and hint that the Sumerians were the world's first beekeepers. But it is believed it was *really* the ancient Egyptians who started the craft of tending to bees and reaping rewards. Wild bee swarms were lured into containers and taken back to the temples and the priests were given the job of tending to the bees. By 2600 B.C., beekeeping was happening and honey was being praised for its versatile uses in medicine, beauty preparations, and trade.[5]

The ancient Egyptians were also known to include honey in cooking, especially for honey cakes, and as offerings to the gods. Jars of honey—which is an excellent preserver—were buried with the pharaohs to sustain them in the afterlife, a practice that was also common in Mesopotamia, where honey was used for its healing health powers.[6]

Sweet Honey Wine of Ancient Myths

The history of mead (honey made into wine) is worth a mention, since its roots go back to rituals of the Celts, Anglo-Saxons, and Vikings. As the legend goes, mead was touted to have healing power. The word "honeymoon" stems from the time when newlyweds indulged in mead for one month following the wedding. As legend has it, if the mead was "proper," a son would be the end result within nine months.

The art of making mead, including adding herbs, began in the Middle Ages. Mixing grape and other fruit wines with this sweet beverage can be traced back to Roman times. As time passed, mead was replaced by beverages such as wine made from grapes or other fruits.

(*Source:* National Honey Board.)

. . . BLOSSOMED TO ANCIENT GREECE AND ROME

Once Egypt paved the way for beekeeping, Greece and Rome were next in line. Aristotle, Hippocrates, and Dioscorides touted honey's magic, noting its amazing remedies, including as a wound salve, a cough medicine, an aid to rid one of body lice, and a cure for earache, ulcers, and even hemorrhoids.

In Greek mythology there are references to honey, with the moniker "the nectar of the gods." After all, it was the Greeks who first noted the flavors of honeys and potpourri of nectar sources. The most beloved honey, from the perspective of the Greeks, was honey that came from thyme—growing on the slopes near Athens. Honey was the only sweetener available in Europe at the time, aside from syrups made from dried fruits, and herbs such as cicely.[7]

The ancient Romans put honey on a pedestal, as the Greeks did. Apicius, a famous gourmand, praised honey in more than half of his recipes, including one for roast dormouse (brushed with honey) and another for honey-baked ham. Both Egyptians and Greeks prized honey as a remarkable food preservative.[8]

The Old Philosopher and the Honey

As the tale goes, Democritus, a Greek philosopher, set his mind on dying at age 110. To achieve this goal he resisted food, day by day. His idea was to limit his food intake until he perished. The glitch was, a festive event was coming and the women in his household coaxed him not to leave Earth until this celebration ended. A translation of the Greet text *Deipnosophistae II* noted: "He was persuaded and ordered a vessel full of honey to be set near him, and in this way he lived for many days with no other support, than the honey; and then some days afterwards when the honey had been taken away, he died."[9]

HONEY SWEETENS UP BRITAIN AND AMERICA

So, there is a trail of evidence that hints that *exactly* when honey made its move from Greece and Rome to the British Isles it was wild bees that deserved credit. Clues have been found on Neolithic pottery remains around 5,000 years back—and beekeeping was likely practiced in England before the Roman invasion. By the 11th century A.D., beekeeping was noted in the Domesday Book list noting the number of hives each landholder owned—to show how important these insects were to mankind.[10]

HONEY SWEETENS THE USA

The European honey bee was brought by man (they did not make the flight themselves) to New England in about 1638. North American natives called these honey bees the white man's flies. Honey was used to prepare food and beverages, to make cement, to preserve fruits, and for medicinal purposes. But tending to honey bees and gathering honey was not perfected as a fine art because of the challenges of beekeeping. Simply put, the intricate extraction of honey was not an easy process for beekeepers or bees.[11]

By the 18th century, however, thanks to the box hive, bees could attach to their honeycombs. But it still wasn't a finished fine art for bees or beekeepers until later in the century. That's when inventors fine-tuned hives so bees could build wax cells and raise their young and store pollen and honey. For centuries honey was eaten as honeycomb, since it was a task to extract the liquid sealed in the cells. This problem was solved when Franz Edler von Hruschka invented the honey extractor.[12]

In the 21st century, beekeeping continued to be an art in itself and the attraction was a mainstay around the globe after its historical roots spread. Major producers of honey include Argentina, China, Mexico, Turkey, the United States, and the Ukraine. These days, much like yesterday, honey, with its healing powers and interest as a natural sweetener and superfood, is in demand by beekeepers and other consumers around the world.

OTHER PAST MEDICAL USES OF HONEY

Historical Users	Ingredients	Uses
Sumerians	River dust mixed with honey and oil	To treat skin ulcers
Egyptians	Honey	To treat open wounds; also used to feed sacred animals
Greeks	Honey	As an offering to the gods and the spirits of the dead
Babylonians	Honey	In medicine (referred to in the Code of Hammurabi)
Sushrutra, a surgeon from India	Honey varietals	For medicinal properties
Charak, another Indian physician	Honey	As tonic and mild laxative
Athenaeus	Honey and bread	To make who ate this for breakfast "free from disease all their lives"

| Ibn Magih, from Arab-Muslim culture | Honey | As a remedy for every illness |
| Chinese | Honey mixed with opium | A therapeutic relief for pain |

(*Source: The Honey Revolution.*)[13]

HONEY MILESTONES

Year	What Happened	What It Did
6000 B.C.	Cave paintings were made in Spain that showed men collecting honey from a bee colony.	They proved honey goes back to ancient times.
2600 B.C.	Beekeeping was established.	Honey began to be used as medicine and for beauty and trade.
30th century B.C.	Honey was used in most households as a sweetening agent.	This showed how much Egyptians valued honey, as it was often used as payment.

Year	What Happened	What It Did
1500s	A book on Chinese medicine, published during the Qin dynasty, touted medicinal uses of honey.	It heightened awareness of honey and health.
1500s	Ibn Magih, prophet, wrote a book, *The Sacred Bee*, discussing honey as a remedy for illness.	It taught people about the healing powers of honey.
1600s	European honey bees were introduced to New England by European settlers.	This encouraged use of honey to prepare food and beverages, to preserve fruits, and for medicinal purposes.
1759	The first English book about honey, by John Hill, was published.	This recognized the healing powers of honey.
1950s	*Folk Medicine*, by D. C. Jarvis, a doctor, was published.	It would make honey popular in the following decades.

Year	What Happened	What It Did
1970s–1980s	Books on bee-keeping and honey were published by Dr. Eva Crane, beekeeper and researcher.	They heightened awareness of honey bees and honey health.

(*Sources:* National Honey Board and South Staffordshire Beekeepers Association.)

I've searched for an all-natural and simple-to-bake cheesecake recipe—and it found me. This is a sweet cheesecake from the Old World, made with five basic, no-nonsense ingredients: plain flour, ricotta cheese, an egg, bay leaves, and clear honey, which was popular in ancient Roman times. I recommend using a different honey varietal each time you make it and every time your Ancient Roman Cheesecake will taste like a first sweet kiss.

Ancient Roman Cheesecake

❖ ❖ ❖

4.2 ounces plain flour	1 beaten egg
4.4 ounces ricotta cheese	Bay leaves
	16 teaspoons clear honey

Sieve the flour into a fairly large bowl.

Beat the cheese until it is soft and stir it into the flour along with the egg. Form a soft dough and divide into four. Form each into a bun and place them on a greased baking tray with a fresh bay leaf underneath each.

Heat the oven to 425°F. Bake for 35–40 minutes until they are golden brown. Warm the honey and place the warm cakes into it [4 teaspoons each] so that they absorb the liquid fully. Allow the cheesecakes to stand for 30 minutes before serving.

(*Source:* Courtesy of Delicious Italy.)

I baked this cheesecake and it's not your typical New York treat—it has a simple, old-world taste. My recommendation is to give it a new-world twist by adding ½ teaspoon vanilla, 1 teaspoon cinnamon, using whole ricotta cheese, adding 1 teaspoon lemon rind, and using your favorite honey type— orange blossom gave it a nice citrusy flavor—and serving it with fresh seasonal berries or dark chocolate curls.

Honey's remarkable powers, from eating to medicinal uses, from biblical times throughout century after century, were touted to have health attributes. Despite the bad rap it has received in the 20th century by nutritionists claiming "it's still a sugar," it's made a turnaround in its acceptance, especially in the past two decades.

Honey, now dubbed as a superfood, has received a thumbs-up by scientists and medical doctors around the globe. In the next chapter, "A Historical Testimony," I'll show you exactly how honey deserves kudos and why it's good enough to snag from the hive like Winnie the Pooh, the storybook bear, did.

UN-BEE-LIEVABLE HEALING HINTS TO CATCH

- ✓ Honey has made its mark in the Bible and is noted for its versatile virtues, including fertility and prosperity for the Promised Land, as a gift and the ultimate healing food.
- ✓ Honey made its name for its amazing powers in Greek mythology and writings of both the Egyptians and Romans.
- ✓ By the 17th century, the European honey bee had been brought by man to America and was touted for its usefulness and remarkable gifts to mankind.
- ✓ Beekeepers and advocates of the healing powers of honey paved the path of healing honey in America in the 1900s.
- ✓ By the mid–20th century and into the 21st century, beekeeping and bees had developed a reputation as one of nature's greatest gifts in America and around the world.

PART 2

NECTAR
OF THE GODS

CHAPTER 3

A Historical Testimony

*There are certain pursuits which, if not wholly
poetic and true, do at least suggest a nobler and
finer relation to nature than we know. The keeping
of bees, for instance.*

—Henry David Thoreau[1]

At 17, like a worker honey bee, I was on a mission. I remember one night I was sheltered under my favorite magnolia tree—the one my father planted in our front yard. I was sitting cross-legged on the grass. Clad in blue jeans and a sleeveless T-shirt and barefoot, I was the poster child of shaggy-haired, restless youth and eager to spread my wings. Sweet memories of my childhood were fading. The garden lacked nurturing. There was talk of my family uprooting to another home, smaller, which to me seemed would be too crowded. It was on this summer evening that I sensed change was in the air.

With big white blossoming flowers above me (they didn't produce nectar or attract the honey bee), I nibbled on a peanut butter and honey sandwich. I refused to eat my mom's liver and onions. It was time to flee like a young honey bee. At first, I took small daily trips, down the California coast to Big Sur—in search of an oasis, a refuge that promised more. I was hardly alone. During the sixties and seventies, like a bee swarm, it was a movement. A new generation of young people traveled from state to state around America and the world in search of a better place to be.

During the seventies, honey bees and beekeepers were also explorers. Pioneers in the bee world understood the wanderlust of the honey bee and its gifts to nature. They knew that honey was versatile and healthful—both inside and outside the body. And these findings have been embraced and are now becoming the latest buzz for the mainstream audience.

HONEY PIONEERS IN THE 20TH CENTURY

I find it intriguing that some of the noteworthy honey producers of the world made history and paved the way for the 21st-century honey companies in California, my native state. Also, what is so interesting is that these pioneers are family run or have ties back to the early 1900s.

The Worldly Bee Lady. On June 12, 1912, Eva Crane was born, and she ended up being a dedicated worker bee as a researcher and author on the subjects of bees and beekeeping. Once a math wizard, she switched her calling to bees and devoted her life to researching bees and traveling around the world. The *New York Times* reported that "Dr. Crane wrote some of the most important books on bees and apiculture."[2]

Crane is most remembered in the honey bee world

for her works, including *Honey: A Comprehensive Survey* (1975), *A Book of Honey* (1980), and *The Archaeology of Beekeeping* (1983). Her writing ended up in two tomes: *Bees and Beekeeping: Science, Practice and World Resources* (1990) and *The World History of Beekeeping and Honey Hunting* (1999). These days, if I had the pleasure to interview her as I did Charles Schulz, another keen observer of mankind and animals, I wonder if I'd capture her interest. I would share my own travel adventures with a knapsack and dog, flittering from state to state like a honey bee.[3]

The Vermont Country Doctor. D. C. Jarvis, like Eva Crane, made his mark in the honey world. This family doctor not only turned to apple cider vinegar, which I noted in my book *The Healing Powers of Vinegar,* to help treat his Vermont patients, but the nectar of the gods was part of his bag of folk remedies to prevent and treat illnesses, too.

The country doctor noted in his classic book *Folk Medicine* that native Vermonters had the "nutritional wisdom of the bee, which goes into the fields and selects the materials for the making of a perfect food." He wrote that the people (not unlike in the 21st century) who knew the food value of honey were more apt to eat it on a regular basis than those who didn't have adequate knowledge of it.

Dr. Jarvis offers many uses for honey. Honey is used for many purposes from athletic nutrition, burns, cramps, cough, and sinusitis to other pesky conditions. (See chapter 11: "Home Remedies from Your Kitchen.")

THE MANUKA HONEY GURU:
DR. PETER MOLAN

Enter Peter Molan, Ph.D., professor of biochemistry at Waikato University, New Zealand. He has been at the forefront of honey research for almost three decades. He heads the university's Honey Research Unit, which is internationally known for its research in the healing powers of honey. In an exclusive interview, I asked Dr. Molan about the future of honey and its place in health and well-being around the globe and in the United States.

Q: *For 27 years, you have been conducting research on the healing powers of manuka honey. What inspired you to delve into this scientific research?*

A: I started the research after a friend, Kerry Simpson, a high school science teacher and keen beekeeper, persuaded me to investigate manuka honey because he had heard of its reputation in New Zealand folk medicine as the best honey to use as an antiseptic.

[Note: Although the manuka tree is used in traditional Maori medicine, there was no honey in New Zealand until European settlers brought honey bees less than two centuries ago. The antibacterial component in manuka honey does not occur in the manuka tree—it is formed as part of a reaction in the ripened honey.]

Q: *What new honey-sensitive bacteria have you discovered that respond to manuka honey?*

A: Manuka honey, even at a concentration as low as 1 percent, stops the growth of campylobacter, bacteria which are a very common cause of diarrhea. It has been found to be effective against a wide range of "superbugs" (bacteria resistant to antibiotics), including MRSA (methicillin-resistant Staphylococcus aureus).

Q: *Currently, manuka honey is FDA approved and available for purchase through the Internet for people in the United States. Do you feel any large drug company in America may produce a manuka honey product and sell it as a prescribed medicine to hospitals and clinics?*

A: Jars of manuka honey on sale in the USA are not approved by the FDA for any therapeutic use, although they are legitimately sold as a food just like any other honey. However, there are various brands of manuka honey on sale with FDA approval for treating wounds. Some are tubes of manuka honey, and some are wound dressings containing manuka honey. All are sterilized products. It is smaller medical companies producing these, but large drug companies are now showing an interest.

Q: *You coined the "UMF (Unique Manuka Factor)" term, which is the antibacterial potency of a given honey. Medical professionals in New Zealand use manuka honey with UMF ratings of 10 or higher. Currently, tests are being done in the U.S. to find out if there is antibacterial potency in other honeys. Which varietals do you feel may make the grade?*

A: I originally devised the term "UMF" for use by any producer of genuine manuka honey to be able to inform consumers that it had the special antibacterial activity found only in manuka honey (and later found to also be in honey from the same type of trees growing in Australia).

It has since been captured as an exclusive brand by some companies, and many producers of the genuine manuka honey are not allowed to use the term. Even the name "unique manuka factor," which I gave to the special activity, has been claimed by the exclusive companies to be their trademark, so I no longer use that name. I, like many honey producers, have for decades used the name "non-peroxide activity" to refer to the special type of antibacterial activity in manuka honey.

The antibacterial activity of other types of honey is due to hydrogen peroxide, which is produced by an enzyme that the bees add to the nectar they collect to make honey. There is an enzyme in body tissues and serum which rapidly destroys hydrogen peroxide. Thus, although honeys other than manuka honey may have a high level of antibacterial activity in laboratory testing, they are unlikely to be as effective on a wound.

Q: *What is the most important study you've had published and why is this groundbreaking?*

A: I don't think any individual publication can be singled out. What has been "groundbreaking" (in that it has got the medical profession using manuka honey) has been the cumulative findings of the effectiveness of manuka honey against wound-infecting bacteria and the explanation of how honey works in other ways as well in getting wounds to heal.

Q: *You have said that at present people are turning to honey when nothing else works. But there are very good grounds for using honey as a therapeutic agent of first choice. Why do you feel U.S. medical professionals are hesitant to use honey as they do in other countries?*

A: I feel the reluctance to use honey comes from lack of knowledge about it, particularly in the USA, where there has been less publicity than in other countries and fewer presentations at wound-care conferences. Especially, I think that not having had presented the scientific rationale for how honey works leaves medical professionals viewing honey as some sort of "snake oil" being marketed.

Q: *And when do you believe the United States will begin using manuka honey in hospitals and clinics?*
A: It already is starting, but on a small scale. I feel that it will not take off on a large scale like has happened in the UK until there are presentations at wound-care conferences explaining the scientific rationale for how honey works (as was done in the UK).

Q: *Meanwhile, can manuka honey be safely ingested by humans if the UMF is less than 10? If so, how much should one consume per day? And what is it best used for in this form? Also, is manuka safe to use as a dressing for our companion animals?*
A: There is a risk to be considered of harmful effects of long-term consumption. I would not consider there to be any significant risk from short-term ingestion, such as treating an infection in the gut. But I do question why anyone would be consuming it regularly, especially the low-activity honey which is unlikely to have any antibacterial effect when diluted by fluid in the gut.

You ask what it is best used for. Wound care, obviously, is a major use (for humans and animals). But this would be with a non-peroxide activity rating above 10. For deep wounds it should be the FDA-approved sterilized products that are used, because otherwise there is a risk of introducing spores of clostridia, which could cause wound botulism and gangrene.

By mouth, treatment of sore throats is a traditional

use of honey. Manuka honey lozenges are now on sale, which should be the most effective way of keeping honey in contact with the throat. A small clinical trial has been conducted on treatment of sore gums (gingivitis) which has indicated a beneficial effect. (I use manuka honey–like toothpaste if I get sore gums.) Another traditional use of honey is for treating stomach ulcers and gastritis (inflammation of the stomach). There has been no established dose for this, but people commonly take a heaped teaspoonful. Some other treatments for which I am getting reports of good results are for eye infections, ear infections, and nasal sinus infections.

For more information, log on to the Web site of the Honey Research Unit of the University of Waikato: http://bio.waikato.ac.nz/honey/

CATCHING UP WITH HONEY MAKERS

When I began my exploration to discover who's who in the honey world I learned quickly that there wasn't a ready-made list compiled of top companies like there is for leading chocolate producers. I followed a path paved by worldly beekeepers that led me to a handful of top honey companies and packers in the United States— the top queen bees in America, which include Sue Bee®, Golden Heritage Foods, and Adee Honey Farms.

Other workers that lead the global honey market, according to Global Industry Analysts, Inc., "include Bee Maid, Billy Bee Honey, Capilano Honey, Comvita Limited, Dabur India Limited, Dutch Gold Honey, Inc., Golden Acres Honey, Hebei Wuqiao Mtl Co., Ltd., Odem International, Inc., Rowse Honey Ltd, Shriro Pvt Ltd., . . . and Yanbian Baolixang Beekeeping Co., Ltd, among others."[4]

During my at-home trek through the honey world, I found a tier of like-minded hardworking down-to-earth people in the honey production world. There are the beekeepers or producers and packers (who fill the glass jars and ship them off themselves to corporate food processors, such as General Mills or Kraft Foods). And there are sideliners or mom-and-pop outlets that make a part-time living from selling bee products. (Go to chapter 14 to find out more about the busy bees and their workers.)

FARMERS' AND MAN'S BEST FRIEND: THE HONEY BEE

Beekeepers also supplement their income by renting out bees for pollination of crops—and this requires travel for both beekeepers and bees, a whole lot of hard work, effort, and time. It's a challenge to pinpoint exactly how many commercial beekeepers are working in the United States, but at least 1,000 seem to be hard at work. It's becoming harder for commercial beekeepers to make a living because of obstacles, whether it is Mother Nature's wrath or the colony collapse phenomenon—when bees die off.

Despite the ups and downs for both the honey bee and the beekeeper, many of the beekeepers, big and small, go back generations and are dedicated workers like their bees, which makes their history fascinating with its roots to the honey bee, past and present.

Sioux Bee / Sue Bee®: In 1921, five beekeepers located near Sioux City, Iowa, got together and formed the Sioux Honey Association. They shared equipment, marketing, and processing facilities. Sue Bee Honey® was born. The rest is history.

In the early days, honey was marketed under the "Sioux Bee" label. Then in 1964 the name was changed to "Sue Bee" because it's easier to pronounce. Later, other lines of honey were added, including the Clover Maid, Aunt Sue, Nature Pure, and Northern American brands. Collectively, around 40 million pounds of honey are produced each year. Sue Bee Honey® is processed in plants located in Sioux City, Iowa; Anaheim, California; and Elizabeth, North Carolina.

These days, Sue Bee®'s global presence extends to the Middle East, the Far East, Europe, and South and Central America and it continues to be a leader in the honey industry.

Golden Heritage Foods: Back in March 2002, with the combining of assets of Barkman Honey Company located in Hillsboro, Kansas, and Stoller's Honey in Latty, Ohio, Golden Heritage Foods was established.

Barkman's and Stoller's similar values, backgrounds in beekeeping and honey packaging, experience, and determination to be the leaders in the honey industry drew these two companies together. Golden Heritage Foods (the company headquarters are located in Hillsboro) is now the number two leader of branded retail honey sales and is the top provider of honey in the U.S. to the food service industry.

Move Over, Honey Bees:
Meet the Honey Man

Who in the bee world was smitten by the sacred honey bee at an early age and followed his heart and the bees for decades? Meet Ted Dennard, the founder of the Savannah Bee Company. He has followed fate and his heart to spin a sweet life for himself and others around the globe.

As the story goes, Ted, a young blond-headed kid, was helping his dad work on his forest retreat in coastal Georgia. The Savannah Bee Company took root when an old battered pickup truck swarming with bees rattled into Ted's life. An elderly man stepped out of the truck with bees crawling all over him.

"Roy Hightower's my name and I've been looking far and wide for an ideal honey-making spot. If you let me put my hives here, I'll introduce you to the marvelous world of honeybees."

At first, thousands of bees buzzing around Ted's head caused more fear than pleasure. The thought of stinging insects all over was almost unbearable. Concentrating on the hum of the bees and their fascinating matriarchal world helped him dismiss outside distractions and his inner fears in a Zen-like fashion.

Old Roy twirled a frame of honeycomb before Ted's eyes so that the sunlight flashed through the honey like nature's stained glass. The intricately patterned, multicolored cells of honey appeared as a window to the honey bee's world. Roy cautioned, "Son, I have to warn you that these bees become a way of life." And so they did.

Ted's university years found him attending Sewanee and living in a cabin rented from a retired minister who, coincidentally, happened to be an avid beekeeper. He once told Ted, "If you study these bees, you can see the hand of God in all that they do." Following Ted's graduation, the U.S. Peace Corps chose him to teach beekeeping in Jamaica. Two years later, upon moving back to the Georgia coast, he learned that the world's two finest honeys (tupelo and sourwood) originated in Georgia. That encouraged him to produce as much of that honey as possible and pursue a dream.

These days, more than two decades after Old Roy passed on to that flower field in the sky, Ted finds himself rattling around in an old truck filled with bees. He spends most of his time in the honey workshop, but when he tends the beehives in deep forested river basins and lush mountain valleys his thoughts go to Roy—the one who introduced Ted to the honey bee.

Meanwhile, Savannah Bee Company products are sold in at least 2,000 stores, and they have sold their honey around the world, including Australia, Canada, Dubai, and Japan. Over the years, Ted has built relationships with beekeepers all over the world: "I buy honey from most of them every year. I also pay them a premium price so they always sell me their best," he says. And yes, the grown-up honey entrepreneur with 25 honey bee colonies of his own uses honey (including acacia and tupelo) in his coffee every morning and in his tea in the afternoon.

So, as Roy the beekeeper cautioned the boy from Georgia, bees indeed would pave a life for Ted, who is thankful for that chance meeting on our little road, and to the honey bee.

OTHER 20TH-TO-21ST-CENTURY HEALTH MILESTONES

It is no surprise that in the 20th century honey was a popular business as it swept the nation and world with its gifts from the honey bee, including its health benefits.

Year	What Happened	Author/Doctor/ Company
1952	*The Nature Doctor*, a classic, was published.	Swiss naturopath Alfred Vogel who recommends honey with echinacea for cuts and wounds
1957	The model of the original honey invented.	Ralph and Luella Gamber, founders of Dutch Gold Honey
1970s	Honey was popularized by a Vermont doctor's best-selling book, *Folk Medicine*, and honey prices skyrocketed.	Dr. D. C. Jarvis

Year	What Happened	Author/Doctor/Company
1975	*Honey: A Comprehensive Survey*, the most significant review of honey ever published, was written by a researcher and author on the subject of bees.	Eva Crane
1994	*Health and the Honey Bee* was penned by a beekeeper and apitherapist who used bee venom to treat patients with arthritis, multiple sclerosis, and other disorders.	Charles Mraz
2000	Presentation about apitherapy was made by an apriculturist at an international bee research association conference in Thailand.	Naomi M. Saville
2010	Groundbreaking research was done on honey, especially manuka, in New Zealand.	Peter Molan, Ph.D.

(*Source:* South Staffordshire Beekeepers Association.)

Honey Is Timeless

Past and present, honey is a food that stimulates the minds of entrepreneurs and creative artisans in America and around the world. Honey and its health benefits were making the news in the late 20th century and continue to do so in the 21st century. And it's not uncommon to find folks in the honey world to enable you to savor the goods they produce. That means recipes that work with honey are part of their life, like this one.

Ted's Savannah Bee Grill Honey Salmon

❖ ❖ ❖

1 pound fresh salmon filet	2 teaspoons Dijon mustard
2 tablespoons white wine vinegar	2 teaspoons Savannah Bee Company Grill Honey
1 tablespoon lemon juice	Fresh rosemary
1 tablespoon olive oil	Salt
	Black pepper

Preheat grill to 350°F. Prepare grilling planks according to directions on package. Make slits in salmon (along the grain) every

1 to 2 inches. Pour vinegar and lemon juice over salmon filet, turning to coat both sides.

Mix olive oil, mustard, and Savannah Bee Company Grill Honey in a small pan over low heat, blending mixture into an emulsion. Pour half of the mixture over fish, turning to coat.

Strip the leaves of the rosemary and roughly chop to release the oils. Gently push rosemary into the slits on the filet.

Heat the plank on the grill for 5 minutes and turn the warm side up. Place fish skin side down on the plank. Pour remaining mixture over the top and close grill. When salmon reaches an internal temperature of 135–145° (about 15 minutes), drizzle Savannah Bee Company Grill Honey liberally over the top and turn up the heat to 450°. After 1–2 minutes pull salmon out and let stand for 5 minutes under foil tent before serving.

(*Courtesy:* Savannah Bee Company.)

Now that I've put honey, nature's sweetest superfood, on the table, it's time to scrutinize its healthful ingredients like it's a frog (dedicated to budding scientists) on a slab in high school biology class. (As a sensitive, devout animal lover, I skipped class on dissection day.)

So, what exactly makes honey a superfood—or is it another added sugar (as some nutritionists claim it to be) that we should stay clear of because it will make us fat and lead to heart woes? I tackle this controversial nutrition topic in the next chapter.

UN-BEE-LIEVABLE HEALING HINTS TO CATCH

- ✓ The United States is a hot spot for honey packers and producers, and its climate and health-conscious nuts and foodies as well as tourists enjoy the progressive honey highlights.
- ✓ Old-time honey companies, including Sue Bee® and Golden Heritage, have held and are holding their place in the global honey industry, past and present.
- ✓ Other well-known major honey companies have made their name in both the 20th and 21st centuries.
- ✓ California's honey packers and producers are touted for their honey products, but they are also praised for their honey bees and pollination services to keep agriculture, including almond production, a thriving industry.
- ✓ While honey producers are busy working in the honey industry, medical doctors, scientists, authors, and health-conscious consumers are aware of the growing trend of the healing powers of honey.
- ✓ The honey industry in the 21st century has captured a worldwide audience because honey's back-to-nature goodness is versatile and promises healing powers for ailments and diseases.

Where Are the Secret Ingredients?

*The only reason for being a bee that I know of is
making honey . . . and the only reason for making
honey is so I can eat it.*
　　　　—Winnie the Pooh in A. A. Milne's
　　　　　　The House at Pooh Corner[1]

At 21, a Californian with a honey bee–like wanderlust, I
thought about joining the Peace Corps or armed services with the promise of travel and to be with other
people—like busy bees in a hive. But I sensed I was different from a worker bee. My travels across America
happened with my own two feet, two arms, and one
thumb. I set out to do just that as a human bee—go
astray from a swarm like a lone honey bee.

One day I gathered up one sleeping bag and a knapsack stuffed with road-friendly foods, including granola
bars and peanut butter. I fled Northern California and
headed south toward Interstate 10. My first goal was
Florida—the Sunshine State, with beaches, palm trees,

and flowers. Naïve like a house bee, I wasn't ready for the world full of pests, nature's wrath (from blizzards to windstorms), and man-made challenges.

Soda and BIT-O-HONEY bars were often the staples of my diet, which lacked nutrition. "California Butterfly"—an insect like the honey bee that also seeks sweet nectar—was the moniker I embraced. During my road adventure, little did I know that honey—not white sugar, which I was eating—was getting kudos from progressive medical experts and health nuts. Some nutritionists and doctors played down the good-for-you nutrients in this liquid gold "cure-all." But there are folks around the world who did and still do believe honey is as good as gold.

These days, in the 21st century, humans are reaping the nutritional rewards of honey, but that doesn't mean the golden liquid is full of nutrients in small amounts. Here's what I found out:

Nutrition Facts:	
Serving Size: 1 Tablespoon (21 g)	
Servings Per Container: 22	
Amount per Serving:	
Calories: 64	
Total Fat: 0 g	
Sodium: 0 g	
Total Carbohydrate: 17 g	
Sugars: 16 g	
Protein: 0 g	

(*Source:* National Honey Board.)

When you look at a honey's product label, it appears to be a health nut's dream come true: The food contains no fat, no cholesterol, and no sodium. But the fact remains, all is not perfect, according to nutritionists, who are quick to point out a large portion of the calories in this superfood comes from sugars—culprits that may lead to heart disease and obesity.

One dietitian told me point-blank that she had no positive words to say about honey. But I argued, "There are tons of anecdotal evidence, studies from countries abroad, and medical experts who do tout the golden liquid." She stuck to her words: "It's sugar, no better, no worse, than other added sugars." Dazed and confused, I went straight to the honey-savvy nutritional gurus who are aware of the sweet stuff in the ancient liquid gold. Studying the nutrition facts for honey is similar to analyzing vinegars—they differ from source to source and company to company, and the bigger the measurements, the more nutrients you'll find.

More Honey, Please

339 grams (one cup) contain:
14 milligrams sodium
279.34 grams carbohydrate
0.7 gram dietary fiber
278.39 grams sugars
1.02 grams protein
1.7 milligrams vitamin C
20 milligrams calcium
1.42 milligrams iron
7 milligrams magnesium
14 milligrams phosphorus
176 milligrams potassium

0.75 milligrams zinc
23.7 milligrams fluoride
2.7 milligrams selenium

Other nutrients: riboflavin, niacin, pantothenic acid, vitamin B$_6$, folate, choline, betaine, amino acids.

Apparently, more honey equals more nutrients. One cup contains more than 1,031 calories, but zero saturated fat, trans fat, or cholesterol.

(*Source:* USDA National Nutrient Database for Standard Reference, 2009.)

It's the Antioxidant Power

Honey wizards such as *SuperFoods HealthStyle* co-author Steven G. Pratt, M.D., note that honey contains at least 181 known substances, nutrients, such as amino acids, carbohydrates (natural sugars), as well as trace enzymes, minerals (including calcium, fluoride, iron, magnesium, phosphorus, and selenium), vitamins (including vitamin C, folate, and choline), and water. But the vitamins and minerals aren't the highlight of honey's healing powers.[2]

As I noted in chapter 1: "The Power of Honey," honey is antioxidant rich and that's where the real power lies, no ifs, ands, or buts about it. We're talking mighty bioflavonoids, flavonoids, and phenolic acids, which act as disease-fighting antioxidants—the good guys that help to keep your body healthy and stall Father Time. It is the darker honeys, like quality dark chocolate, that contain more antioxidants—and that's what really accounts for honey's healing powers. But that's not all. . . .

Here's proof: It's been proven in past studies—more than one—by scientists that for people, not rats, eating honey raises blood levels of good-for-you antioxidants. A connection was made with 25 healthy men who drank plain water or water with buckwheat honey. Those who chose the honey concoction had a 7 percent increase in their antioxidant levels.[3]

To Be 100 Percent Pure Honey— or Not?

People in the honey bee world, including the National Honey Board, know that the honey they see in some grocery stores and dollar stores may not be 100 percent pure but instead be "adulterated" (contaminated with tainted elements). This fact is upsetting to people because not only are we not getting what we pay for, but we also are being duped, as often the honey is tainted with unhealthful, cheaper ingredients such as antibiotics. This ordeal is making headlines in the news more rather than less and it's causing concern for both consumers and beekeepers.

All-natural, 100 percent pure honey will have *one* ingredient listed on the nutrition label: *honey*. Imitation honeys, much like quality imitation dark chocolate, are not a laughing matter in the real world. That means trouble lies ahead for real honey lovers who want to "save the endangered honey bee." Honey-flavored syrups, or honey that's diluted with other ingredients, are becoming more commonplace and being sold to the unaware consumer. To be sure you get the pure golden food of the gods, check the label.

(*Source:* National Honey Board.)

HONEY IS NOT JUST ANOTHER SWEETENER

During my trek through Honeyland, the words "honey is still a sugar" echoed from one nutritionist to another—it was a domino effect, sort of. I sensed that many of these food experts did not go the distance to learn about the antioxidant value of honey varietals in the United States and around the world. Honey, with all its virtues, is not just a miracle fly-by-night snack that has made the news. It's real food with real merit.

The Honey Revolution co-author Ron Fessenden, M.D., like me, is sharing the buzz about healing honey: "When compared to table sugar (sucrose) or high fructose corn syrup (HFCS), honey contains nearly the same ration of fructose and glucose." However, adds the honey guru, "Honey contains dozens of different substances, which makes it more like fruit than sugar." And since sugar and HFCS are simpler compounds by comparison, containing only glucose and fructose, honey is a standout sweetener and functional food.

Many Tahoe summers ago, I had a thing for walking outdoors on a hot day to visit a local ice-cream store to buy a cool shake or smoothie. My reward would be enhanced fitness, a golden tan, and an ice-cold beverage to sip on the way home. One day I did research on the

Internet and discovered the ingredients in the smoothie I had savored.

I dumped my habit of buying prepared beverages; it was my last smoothie full of sugar, corn syrup, artificial flavors, concentrated fruit juices, dyes, and stuff I can't pronounce. Worse, the bad buzz is that the words "high-fructose corn syrup" may be changed to "corn sugar" on food labels.

So, making and sipping do-it-yourself cool beverages—with pure honey—was a learning experience. And it brought back memories to when I wrote about smoothies for *Woman's World* magazine. The nutritionists who made up those concoctions used fat-free ingredients and other stuff that wasn't fresh and natural. Homemade smoothies can be sweet and should be real.

HONEY TERMS AT A GLANCE

Other products you buy that contain honey often use words on the product nutrition label that might make you scratch your head and look around for a translator in need of decoding what you're looking at and really getting.

Dried Honey is dehydrated over very high heat and mixed with starches or sugars to keep it flowing.

Flavored/Fruited Honey has either fruit, coloring, or flavoring.

Kosher Honey is produced, processed, and packaged according to Jewish dietary regulations and certified by a kosher organization.

Organic Honey is produced, processed, and packaged according to USDA regulations on organic products and certified by a USDA agency or organization.

So How Much Honey Is Too Much?

Here I sit mulling over the contents of my pantry and wondering, *How many spoonfuls can I enjoy each day?* Well, I made the rounds to book authors, medical doctors, and registered dietitians, and the American Heart Association recommends 6 teaspoons (about 100 calories) of added sugar daily for women, no more than 9 teaspoons for men. Translate that number to honey—an added sugar—and 5 teaspoons of honey for women, 8 teaspoons of honey for men, is just about right.

Refer to chapter 5: "Honey, You're Amazing!" to discover how honey is the sweetener of choice for diabetics and other people who want to stay heart-healthy and lean and live longer.

While I'm still pondering those smoothies I sipped, this is a good time to share an all-natural do-it-yourself bee beverage I whipped up and enjoyed. Using all-natural ingredients makes a big difference in taste and appreciation of what you're putting into your body.

Worker Bee Mocha Shake

❖ ❖ ❖

½ cup 2 percent organic milk
½–¾ cup all-natural Häagen-Dazs honey vanilla ice cream
3 tablespoons brewed coffee

1 tablespoon organic gourmet chocolate honey or fudge sauce sweetened with honey
4 small ice cubes

In a blender, mix milk, ice cream, coffee, and chocolate sauce. Add ice cubes and blend till smooth. Pour into a parfait glass and sip with a straw. Serves one.

It doesn't take a rocket scientist to tell you that honey is a functional food with health-boosting nutrients—especially its mighty antioxidants. So, the question is: How does this ancient essential elixir that is available to us in the modern day help your body inside and outside to prevent disease? Scientists, medical doctors, nutritionists, and beekeepers told me everything I wanted to know and more about how honey heals, and you'll find out its secret healing powers in the next chapter.

UN-BEE-LIEVABLE HEALING HINTS TO CATCH

- ✓ In the 21st century, honey is touted for its vitamins, minerals, and antioxidants.
- ✓ Honey is praised for its healthy sweetener virtues: It has no fat, no cholesterol, and no sodium.
- ✓ Nutritionists in the United States disagree about the health virtues of honey just as they do about dark chocolate.
- ✓ The quality of honey matters. It's real, raw, unprocessed, unheated, unfiltered honey—straight from the hive—that is the superfood nutritionists applaud.
- ✓ It's pure honey—without honey-flavored syrups or high-fructose corn syrup—that consumers want to purchase and consume.

✓ Honey products are processed in different ways, from kosher to organic, to satisfy all honey lovers.

✓ Honey is a sweetener and is recommended to incorporate in the daily diet but in moderation, like chocolate.

✓ The pairing of quality honey with nutrient-rich antioxidant foods can help lower the risk of developing heart disease, diabetes, and cancer.

CHAPTER 5

Honey, You're Amazing!

The secret of my health is applying honey
inside and oil outside.
— Democritus, contemporary of
Hippocrates[1]

As I traveled through the Mojave Desert and Arizona, I felt calm in a warm comfort zone with sagebrush and wildflowers. Then I was tested in a land of strangers. Once I hit Texas there was no turning back. The West Coast granola girl who survived on foods from salads and bean sprouts to fruit and honey was alone like a forager bee without its colony in foreign territory.

One morning I woke up from sleeping outdoors at a desolate campground. I was used to eating fresh fruit, hot tea, and honey. I must have appeared like a disoriented honey bee in search of its swarm. A stranger came to my rescue. A truck driver gave me a lift to a roadside restaurant. I was welcomed with southern hospitality. But the menu items were culture shock. Hominy, grits, biscuits, butter, and bacon were the staples. When I asked the waitress, "Do you have plain yogurt, and fresh?" her eyes met mine. There was a pregnant pause. I felt like a green creature from outer space. I heard her words loud and clear in a southern accent: "Say what, now?" I ended up nibbling on strange breakfast foods but savored and stocked up on the biscuits drizzled with honey.

I learned throughout my time on the road that eating simple and fresh produce is key to staying healthy—thanks to our hardworking pollinating honey bees. But sometimes during the road trip I didn't have a choice. I ate candy bars and soda like a bee eating a mix of sugary foods.

In the 21st century, I believe it's a diet of all-natural foods, Mother Nature's finest, that is key to keeping healthy and staving off heart disease, high blood pressure, type 2 diabetes, and other culprits. Research shows the connection of a healthy diet and lifestyle to good health. And yes! Yes, honey—an added sugar—can and does help fight and even prevent health problems. Here's the health buzz about healing honey.

SO, HOW DOES HONEY HEAL, ANYHOW?

While honey varietals do have their individual healing properties, honey itself has many healing powers.

It's the antioxidants: These enzymes work both inside the body and outside the body to help stave off disease and the aging process.

It's the power of osmosis: Because of the high-sugar, low-moisture content of honey, it creates an osmotic effect, drawing liquid out of anything that comes into contact with it—such as bacteria, which dries up.

It's acidic: Like vinegar, honey is acidic (its pH is between 3 and 4, about the same as orange juice and not as strong as vinegar), which creates an unfriendly environment for bacteria.

It's got hydrogen peroxide: Because of this antiseptic (remember our moms put this clear liquid on our wounds when we were kids to help get rid of germs), honey has antibacterial benefits and is a gentle healer.

HEAL YOURSELF, HONEY

For thousands of years people in the European countries, from Greece and Italy to France, have shared lower rates of obesity and heart disease than people elsewhere. The consensus is that a healthy diet and lifestyle—which includes dark honey and dark chocolate—is the common thread.

The buzz is, honey heals. Anecdotal evidence, past and present day, and studies in countries other than the United States show the healing powers of honey and how it may help to lower the risk of developing health problems, including heart disease, diabetes, and even some cancers, too. Some doctors in the United States are turning sweet on healing honey. Here, take a peek at what's going on in the world of honey and health.

HONEY AND THE BIG C

According to scientific research, cancer-fighting antioxidants that are found in dark honeys may help lower the risk of developing some cancers. But it's the combination of an antioxidant-rich diet with vegetables and fruits and a healthy lifestyle that may keep cancer at bay—not honey as a quick fix.

How Honey Works: Still, research is in the works to find out if the hardworking honey bees are the key to helping humans lower the risk of developing cancer. "Croatian researchers found significantly decreased tumor growth and spreading of the cancer in mice when honey was ingested orally or by injection. Honey was found to be an effective agent for inhibiting the growth of bladder cancer," *101 Optimal Life Foods* author David Grotto, R.D., L.D.N., told me. We both discovered that research also has shown that honey applied to sores reduced discomfort in people enduring cancer treatment, which can lead to side effects such as sores in the inside of the mouth. But honey may be able to do more than be used in rat research and postcancer treatments.

Did you know . . . honey is a potent stimulant of the immune system in humans? It is, reveals *The Honey Revolution* doctor Ron Fessenden, who says honey may inhibit metabolic stress, reducing the production of the hormone cortisol—one of the bad guys that affect our immune system in a bad way. And yes, a good immune response is a good way to lower your odds of having to face cancers, which can be life threatening.

Enter bee propolis. In chapter 1, I introduced this "bee glue" that is showing its stuff to the world. For centuries propolis has been praised as an antiviral and cell regeneration stimulant. Propolis contains bioflavonoids and antioxidants. "More than 300 compounds have been identified in propolis samples, including polyphenols, and many of these compounds have surprising protective effects," notes *The 150 Healthiest Foods on Earth* author Dr. Jonny Bowden.[2]

Scientific articles are published around the world that link infection-fighting properties with propolis—a honey bee's gift to mankind. One compound from bee glue—caffeic acid phenethyl ester (CAPE)—is touted for its immune-boosting powers and is believed to stop the growth of tumor cells. Propolis has also been noticed for its ability to stimulate antibody production, making it an immune-system booster.[3]

The buzz about a Malaysian honey with its potential cancer-fighting powers also caught my eye. According to research conducted at the Universiti Sains Malaysia, Kelantan, dozens of studies showed that tualang honey has antioxidant properties that can halt the growth of certain cancer cells.[4]

Acacia honey, like the Malaysian variety, also has antioxidant properties. Italian researchers discovered chrysin, a natural flavone, in this honey varietal that shows promise as an antitumor agent. Further research is needed to prove that it can be useful as a medicine to help real humans, not just passing tests with human cells with flying colors.

Not only are propolis and Malaysian honey on the table for further research to keep cancer at bay, but bee venom just might be another cancer fighter: "Research published in the FASEB Journal's current [August 2010] issue demonstrates that a key ingredient in the toxic venom released during bee stings can be used as a transporter agent to more effectively deliver drugs or diagnostic dyes to identify and fight tumors."[5]

What You Can Do: No, eating a spoonful of honey or taking propolis each day is not the cure-all for keeping cancer at bay for a lifetime—but it can't hurt to incorporate honey into your diet. Also, eating at least 5 servings of fruits and vegetables per day (recommended by the American Cancer Society) may help keep you cancer free, too. And superfood honey—the raw, darker antioxidant-rich types, such as buckwheat—paired with anticancer superfoods can be the beginning of an arsenal for you to keep the big "C" out of your life.

HONEY FIGHTS FAT

Nutritionists who believe honey is just another sugar will tell you that honey is not going to be a fat-burning miracle worker. Not true.

Cooking and baking, for instance, will allow you to use less honey than sugar because honey is sweeter. Also, if you have a sweet tooth and are craving sweets, including cakes, cookies, and candies, taking a teaspoon of honey will satisfy your desire to overindulge in sweets laden with sugar that'll pack on unwanted calories that come with plenty of fat, sodium, and cholesterol. But sweet, pure honey contains no fat, no sodium, and no cholesterol. One teaspoon is a mere 21 calories. Plus, it's been proven that honey provides an instant energy boost, so you are more apt to get a move on and burn more calories the way athletes do.

How Honey Works: Honey can work to burn fat, reveal Mike and Stuart McInnes, authors of *The Hibernation Diet*. They believe fueling up your liver before bed with 1 or 2 tablespoons of honey will optimize fat-burning potential. "During sleep, our body uses fat for energy during rest and recovery. For this to occur, our liver must be adequately stocked with fuel reserves to get through the eight-hour fast."[6]

Honey may be your best friend forever to fight fat, but what about bee pollen to curb your appetite? Bee pollen may also help you to blast fat, according to honey-savvy holistic nutritionists such as Canada-based Angela Ysseldyk (www.beepollenbuzz.com). Credit goes to its lecithin (bee pollen is rich in it), she explains, because it is a fat emulsifier and having adequate amounts of it in your system may help the fat-burning process.

What You Can Do: While bee pollen may help fight body fat, liquid honey with bee pollen in it may be the sweetest way to go. (I tried tasting bee pollen in honey and it's not easy to swallow unless you're a honey bee. Before bedtime take a spoonful of honey. Nutritionists recommend 1 tablespoon in a variety of ways, including putting it into a cup of tea or a smoothie, on a slice of toast, or into a pot of low-fat plain yogurt.

HONEY AND VINEGAR: THE FABULOUS FAT BURNERS

Not only can honey help burn fat, but its counterpart apple cider vinegar can help you to fight fat, too. Apple cider vinegar is rich in fiber and bloat-busting potassium, and it's got another fat fighter that works. Acetic acid, the main ingredient in vinegar, has long been believed by vinegar lovers to rev up metabolism and to dissolve fat. What's more, sweet honey can sweeten bloat-busting fruit or a glass of water with vinegar and help you to burn fat faster and get a flatter tummy.

Remember, dark honey is best. It has only 21 calories per teaspoon. It has no fat. It has no sodium. It has no cholesterol. It gives you energy, so you can exercise to burn off more calories. But there's more to this diet plan than vinegar and honey.

Complex Carbs: Research shows that carbohydrates play a big role in revving up your calorie-burning power. That's because the body has to work harder to process carbs than it does to process fats. Smart carb choices include fiber-rich fruits and vegetables. Fiber contains zero calories, but its bulk deceives the brain into thinking we're getting them.

Lean Protein–Rich Foods: To keep your metabolism up, include protein-rich foods (skinless chicken and turkey, fish, and egg whites) with your complex carbs at meals. It's the balance of carbs and proteins that boosts the thermogenic factor of the meal. This can help the body produce heat and burn more calories. Plus, low-fat protein-rich foods, like these, can curb hunger pains.

Good Fats: You can indulge in good fats, like extra virgin olive oil, in moderation. Not only is olive oil a healthful fat, but it can make vegetables taste better with vinegar and spices and it can help fill you up also.

THE TWO-DAY HONEY AND VINEGAR DIET

This quickie fat-fighting jump-start two-day meal plan was designed by New Jersey–based Toni Gerbino. It is a classic diet she created for me more than a decade ago, to which she gave a new, improved sweet 21st-century update.

"It's the synergy of the foods" that makes this diet plan work, says the diet guru. "It's not about how much you eat; it's about what you're eating." That means you don't have to count calories. As a prefall detox cleanse, I tried it (again) and my tummy was flat on day three. You can lose up to 6 pounds in two days (it varies depending on your individual size) and feel more energized and ready to start following a healthful diet plan like the Mediterranean diet. (Refer to chapter 6: "The Mediterranean Sweetener.")

Breakfast:
    Fresh seasonal berries or half grapefruit (with 1 teaspoon honey)
    Egg whites

Lunch:
    4 ounces fresh white meat turkey or chicken
    Dark leafy greens with dressing made of fresh parsley, 1 tablespoon each extra virgin olive oil and apple cider vinegar, and spices to taste
    1 cup fresh seasonal berries or half a grapefruit (with 1 teaspoon honey)

Dinner:
    6–8 ounces fresh flounder, sole, or salmon
    Asparagus with lemon, apple cider vinegar, and parsley
    1 cup fresh seasonal berries or half a grapefruit (with 1 teaspoon honey)

- Drink a minimum of six 8-ounce glasses of water with fresh lemon throughout the day.
- Include fat-fighting green tea three times per day. This fat-burning tea contains norepinephrine, a brain chemical that speeds up your metabolism.
- You may use up to 5 teaspoons of honey each day . . .
- . . . and don't forget fat-burning raw apple cider vinegar (1 to 3 teaspoons per day). It's tastier with honey in hot tea or on vegetables with olive oil.
- Take a multivitamin mineral supplement.
- Check with your doctor before starting this or any diet.

HEARTY CHUNKS OF HONEY

A healthful diet and lifestyle is part of the arsenal to beat the battle of the bulge, which can often be linked sooner rather than later to heart disease—still America's number one killer for both men and women, according to the American Heart Association.

Heart-healthy honey may help you to lower blood pressure and regulate cholesterol by reducing the bad kind (LDL) while maintaining the good kind (HDL).

High Blood Pressure

It's the total heart-healthy diet and healthy lifestyle package that may help keep blood pressure numbers normal—not *just* honey. But honey can be a good thing for your heart.

How Honey Works: It's time you can say, "Please pass the honey," rather than pass on the sweet stuff, because its oligosaccharides—good-for-you antioxidants—may help reduce blood pressure. But that's not all. . . .

The Honey Revolution author Fessenden links sleep deprivation and elevated blood pressure. If you're not getting adequate zzz's it can lead to hypertension, since you're not allowing your body to get its needed rest and rejuvenation. That's why consuming honey before bedtime is heart-healthy, because it "reduces the release of adrenaline, a catecholamine that raises blood pressure and heart rate," says Fessenden. "Longer sleep means a reduced risk for hypertension."[7]

What You Can Do: Try eating 1 teaspoon of honey before bedtime. Pairing it with a cup of milk or herbal tea will increase the odds of you getting seven to eight hours of sleep and keeping those BP numbers at 120/80—and lower.

And chances are, if you have high blood pressure you may have high cholesterol, too.

Cholesterol Ups and Downs

In adults, total cholesterol levels of 240 milligrams or higher are considered high risk and levels from 200 to 239 are considered borderline high risk, according to the AHA. Your triglyceride level should not be more than 150. Research proves that polyphenols—like the kind found in honey—can help you stay heart-healthy. Research shows bee foods may also have a positive benefit on the heart.

How Honey Works: A small study in Japan showed that royal jelly supplements lower cholesterol levels in humans. The scientists studied the effects on cholesterol and triglycerides. Several people took 6 grams a day of a royal jelly supplement for four weeks. Their total cholesterol and low-density LDL "bad" cholesterol was much lower than that of those people in the control group who experienced no change in cholesterol levels.[8]

What You Can Do: If you want to lower your cholesterol, you may get help from royal jelly like queen bees do. This bee "caviar" supplies heart-healthy B vitamins, antioxidants C and E, more than a dozen minerals, 18 amino acids, and other key heart helpers. Royal jelly is available at health-food stores. It's sold in a variety of forms, including fresh royal jelly, royal jelly honey (this is what I have, and it is edible in smoothies), and capsules. The recommended dose is 1 to 2 royal jelly capsules daily, says Ray Sahelian, M.D., but he adds that it is difficult to prescribe a specific dosage since each person is different in how they respond.[9] Consult with your health practitioner if you go the royal jelly route. But don't stop there.

The fact is, medical doctors will tell you that the teaming of aging and a sedentary lifestyle with other bad habits (i.e., smoking, overeating) means your risk of high cholesterol and high blood pressure is apt to go up, not down. While 1 to 2 teaspoons of honey multiple times per week may lower your risk of developing heart disease, too, it is the wholesome diet and lifestyle habits (including regular exercise) that can also help you regulate cholesterol levels and blood pressure and keep heart problems at bay—and don't forget the scourge of diabetes.

HONEY AND DIABETES RISK?

According to the American Diabetes Association, more than 18 million Americans have diabetes. An estimated 90 to 95 percent of Americans have type 2, which boomers and elderly people are facing as target groups that might be stung.

How Honey Works: Research shows that honey helps maintain blood-sugar levels in athletes. A study of 39 male and female athletes following a workout ate a protein supplement mixed with a sweetener. Those who ate the supplement sweetened with honey, instead of sugar or maltodextrin, achieved better results. They enjoyed optimal blood-sugar levels for two hours after the workout and experienced better muscle recuperation.[10]

Nutritionists will warn you that honey is still sugar, so if you've blood-sugar issues, proceed with caution. If you check out the glycemic index, honey ranks 62nd, table sugar 64th. The glycemic index measures how your body turns carbohydrates into glucose, triggering an insulin response, explain nutritionists who believe people with diabetes should consume honey in moderation, if at all. If you are diabetic but want to include the golden nectar in your diet, use the good stuff, pure, raw honey.

What You Can Do: Try 1 to 2 teaspoons multiple times a week and avoid added sugars in your diet regime. Also, eating more fiber-rich foods, lowering dietary fat, and exercising regularly help aid in blood-sugar control. People who have type 2 diabetes can usually control the disease by diet and lifestyle changes. To be safe, always check with your health-care provider before making any sweet changes to your daily regime.

LONG LIVE YOU AND YOUR HONEY

Honey has a long shelf life and if you turn to honey for health improvements and health ailments, the golden liquid just may help to extend your longevity. Naturally, if you dodge cancer, diabetes, heart disease, and obesity, this in itself will help you to live a better life, right? And there are people who can tell you that honey is what keeps them going—even after age 100.

What's more, honey proponents believe royal jelly, the stuff that is a key player in the making of the queen bee (the only bee that is fed this creamy thick fluid her entire life), is rich in natural hormones and B vitamins. Because of this food fit for a queen, she lives 40 times longer and is larger than the other bees in the hive. For humans, royal jelly may help increase longevity, provide antiaging benefits, and preserve vitality in the body.

One well-known pioneer of the honey industry at the Comvita Company shows the longevity honey connection at work. At 63, Claude Stratford could be found in his basement at home making and selling bee products. In 1976, he teamed with beekeeper Alan Bougen—two entrepreneurs ready to change the people's ideals of natural health. The duo believed wholeheartedly in the healing powers of bee products, and in the seventies they were the first to export New Zealand manuka honey in a jar. The secret to Claude's longevity may be 2 teaspoons of bee pollen, manuka honey, and olive leaf extract each day.[11]

Speaking of longevity, Wendy Iturrizaga witnessed and documented "the sweet aphrodisiac" at work by observing her neighbors, a retired couple but very active, indulging in the hobbies of cycling and apiculture:

> In their back garden they have several beehives that they take care of with diligence. Every morning very early I can see them from my bedroom window walking up the hill to take care of their beloved bees. After lunch it is almost sure that they will spend the afternoon cycling in the countryside and from what they say, they spend very active nights as well!
>
> The couple who last summer cycled France from north to south confessed to me that they owe their energy to their bees. They systematically consume honey and pollen every day. Honey on toast, pollen and yogurt, honey and crepes, tea and honey. They even make their own jams, breads and biscuits with honey. It is not a surprise my neighbors could manage the Tour de France."[12]

The following recipe was created as part of cholesterol-lowering program for Chicago firefighters. It's quick, simple, and tasty—containing healing foods that include sweet honey.

Firefighter's Honey Muesli

❖ ❖ ❖

1 teaspoon honey
½ cup rolled oats
½ cup skim milk or
    low-fat vanilla soy
    milk

1 ounce mixture of
    almonds, walnuts
    and pistachios
⅛ cup mixed
    dried fruit

Mix all ingredients and eat immediately or cover, refrigerate overnight, and eat the next day. Break it down. . . . Calories: 330; Total Fat: 8 grams; Saturated Fat: 1 gram; Cholesterol: 0 milligrams; Sodium: 90 milligrams; Total Carbs: 56 grams; Dietary Fiber: 6 grams; Sugars: 10 grams; Protein: 11 grams.

(*Source:* Dave Grotto, R.D.)

In the next chapter, I'll show you how the traditional Mediterranean diet and its common foods, including honey as a sweetener, continue to get a thumbs-up in medical journals and studies. It's the antideprivation eating and lifestyle habits—regular exercise teamed with both good fats and sweets (including honey!)—that works for me and can work for you.

UN-BEE-LIEVABLE HEALING HINTS TO CATCH

✓ Honey may help boost your quality of life and enhance longevity by staving off age-related diseases.

✓ Healing honey with its powers is acknowledged around the world as a healing medicine.
✓ Honey heals in a variety of ways—antioxidants, osmosis, acidic, and bacterial.
✓ Honey is a fat-burning food because it provides the body with energy to repair cells and burn fat.

HONEY KEEPS THE DOCTOR AWAY

Disease/Condition	How Honey Works
Obesity	The fructose and glucose in antioxidant-rich dark honey satisfy your sweet cravings so overindulgence in fattening and/or sugary foods without nutritional value is easier to avoid.
Heart Disease	Antioxidants in dark honey help to lower the risk of high blood pressure and high cholesterol.
Diabetes	Dark honey may cut the amount of "bad" LDL cholesterol in the blood, which may lower the risk of developing type 2 diabetes.

| Cancer | Phenols in dark honey act as disease-fighting anti-oxidants to hinder the cancer process and may reduce certain cancers. |
| Aging | Dark honey in moderation lowers the risk of heart obesity, heart disease, diabetes, and cancer—all diseases that can shorten life span. |

The Mediterranean Sweetener

Tart Words make no Friends: a spoonful of honey will. Catch more flies than Gallon of Vinegar.
—Benjamin Franklin[1]

Like a wayward honey bee in flight, I traveled through the New England states and two provinces—Quebec and Ontario—with my Lhasa apso/Maltese, Tiger. He was sweet and bold. I had rescued the white shaggy-haired pooch in Washington State, where blackberry honey is popular. It was this Bohemian lifestyle—hitching rides with my dog and eating a simple, natural diet (including honey when I could afford it)—that kept me lean and healthy.

With my shaggy-haired canine in tow I headed toward Canada. (I had to smuggle him into the country because I didn't have paperwork that was required.)

Once we crossed the border, the closer to the city we got, the more disoriented I felt, not accustomed to being like a honey bee in a swarm. The locals spoke fluent French. (I did not.) The street signs were foreign and the metric system on food labels confused me. I was lost, but I had my dog that was American.

One night my canine companion and I spent in a forest off the main road. We snuggled up in my sleeping bag. Another creature comfort I enjoyed was the foods I guarded stuffed in my backpack: fresh fruit, nuts, whole-wheat bread, peanut butter—and a jar of clover honey. It was a reality TV show real-life moment when I used my finger to scoop out the creamy butter and gooey honey. And yes, I shared a bit of honey, butter, and bread with Tiger (today reminding me of Cerberus, the three-headed dog who was fed a honey cake).

Tiger and I had cuddled and slept in the backyard of Quebec, on beaches in the Florida Keys amid wildflowers, on an Indian reservation in Arizona, in a cornfield in Kansas, and in the back of a pickup truck under the stars at a motel in Tennessee. From truck stops to national parks, this dog and I were inseparable, like bees and their beekeeper. Tiger was my protector and sounding board. It was comfort foods, honey, peanut butter, and whole-grain crackers from the United States, that didn't spoil, kept me energized—and I shared with my best friend.

And while I didn't know it then, later on as a health author I learned I was eating foods of the Mediterranean diet—heart-healthy honey and peanut butter (in moderation) with a dog that provided heart health benefits, too, by keeping my blood pressure down during stressful and lonely times.

MY BUZZ ON THE MEDITERRANEAN DIET AND HONEY

So, what is the heart-healthy Mediterranean diet, anyhow? There's no one "Mediterranean" diet. As the American Heart Association explains it, at least 16 countries border the Mediterranean Sea. Naturally, diets, including French, Italian, and Spanish, differ in the foods of choice. But the deal is, there still is a common thread in the cuisine of the diets.

That means, if I got my long-awaited trip to Europe (especially France, Greece, and Italy), while the dishes I'd savor would be different, the staples would share similarities. The upside of the Mediterranean diet, notes the AHA, is that folks who eat the average Mediterranean diet (in which more than 50 percent of fat calories come from monounsaturated fat, usually from olive oil) eat less saturated fat than you'll find in the typical American diet. And heart disease in Mediterranean countries is still lower in numbers than in the United States, where it's the number one killer for both women and men. And longevity is still higher in Mediterranean countries.

The AHA believes that these facts may be due to not just the Mediterranean diet but also lifestyle choices, such as getting more physical activity and having a strong social support system. The jury is still out for the AHA before they recommend people follow a Mediterranean diet.

Another food pyramid of interest—author Steven Pratt, M.D.'s SuperFoodsRx HealthStyle Pyramid, has similarities to the Oldways traditional Mediterranean Diet Pyramid. His daily pyramid includes fruits (3–5 servings), vegetables (5–7 servings), whole grains (5–7 servings), non- or low-fat dairy (1–3 servings), fish with bones (1–3 servings), dark green leafy greens (1–3 servings), healthy fats (1–2 servings), and up to 100 calories daily of buckwheat honey—as well as aerobic exercise most days (30–90 minutes) and 8 or more 8-ounce glasses of water.

The SuperfoodsRx Healthstyle Pyramid and Oldways traditional Mediterranean diet and lifestyle can keep you working like a worker bee. If you follow the Mediterranean path, you can keep slim and fit like Frenchwomen can and do because of portion control, minimeals, saying no to deprivation, savoring fresh whole food, and keeping a move on—secrets that work effortlessly.

OLDWAYS TRADITIONAL MEDITERRANEAN DIET

My Mediterranean diet of choice, based on the Mediterranean Oldways pyramid, was created using the most current nutrition research to represent a healthy, traditional Mediterranean diet. It was based on the dietary traditions of Crete, Greece, and southern Italy in 1960. This was a time when the rates of chronic disease among the population there were among the lowest in the world and the adult life expectancy was among the highest.

The diet of the poor people of the southern Mediterranean, which consisted mainly of fruits and vegetables, beans and nuts, healthy grains, fish, olive oil, and a small amount of sweets and red wine, proved to be much more likely to lead to longevity. And it's this plant-based diet that is still praised today around the globe.

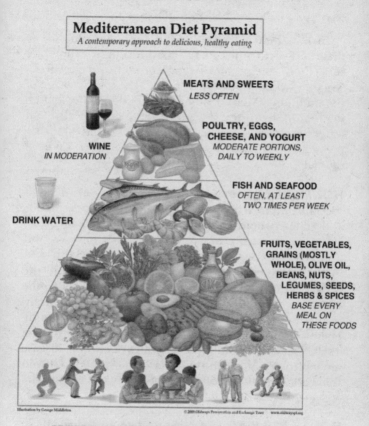

Mediterranean Diet Pyramid
A contemporary approach to delicious, healthy eating

MEATS AND SWEETS
LESS OFTEN

POULTRY, EGGS, CHEESE, AND YOGURT
MODERATE PORTIONS, DAILY TO WEEKLY

WINE
IN MODERATION

FISH AND SEAFOOD
OFTEN, AT LEAST TWO TIMES PER WEEK

DRINK WATER

FRUITS, VEGETABLES, GRAINS (MOSTLY WHOLE), OLIVE OIL, BEANS, NUTS, LEGUMES, SEEDS, HERBS & SPICES
BASE EVERY MEAL ON THESE FOODS

Illustration by George Middleton

© 2009 Oldways Preservation and Exchange Trust www.oldwayspt.org

BE PHYSICALLY ACTIVE; ENJOY MEALS WITH OTHERS

The Bees' Knees Mediterranean Superfoods

In my *Healing Powers* series I push the philosophy that there is no quick fix for good health by eating one superfood—including vinegar, olive oil, and chocolate. Not only would it be boring, but it's the total package of the traditional Mediterranean diet and lifestyle, including honey, that is the golden ticket to good health and longevity. Here's the best of my world with new, improved honey rules I incorporated into my Mediterranean food.

HONEY RULE #1: Go semi-vegan. I eat a plant-based diet, including fruits and vegetables, potatoes, breads and grains (whole grains), beans (I don't like these because they're fuzzy), nuts (I love almonds, cashews, and walnuts), and seeds. But I also incorporate fish and poultry and eggs into my diet on occasion. **Bit o' Honey:** Try drizzling whole-grain bread and nuts with honey.

HONEY RULE #2: Eat fresh foods. If it's seasonally fresh and locally grown I'm there to get my dose of antioxidants. I am Ms. Natural, a produce gal. **Bit o' Honey:** I include all-natural, dark honeys, including buckwheat and manuka, in my diet and lifestyle.

HONEY RULE #3: Use olive oil like an Italian. I use extra virgin olive oil in cooking and baking and on French bread. It is the main fat in my kitchen. I admit that I'll use a bit of European-style butter (especially if I sauté fish or bake scones), but it's EVOO; that's the oil of choice. **Bit o' Honey:** I sometimes use pure maple syrup or organic brown sugar, but sweet honey is the sweetest sweetener you'll find in my pantry.

HONEY RULE #4: Kiss off saturated fat. I aim for a daily total fat amount ranging from about 25 to 35 percent of energy, with saturated fat composing no more than 7 to 8 percent of calories. It's easier to do when you stay clear of meat, butter, and cheese. **Bit o' Honey:** Honey doesn't contain fat, so you can use it to add flavor to foods, in ways such as drizzling it on a whole-grain muffin or pancakes, rather than using high-fat butter.

HONEY RULE #5: Include cheese and yogurt. No need to stay clear of goat cheese or Greek yogurt, but I do go for low-fat varieties. **Bit o' Honey:** Instead of eating yogurt infused with artificial fruits and sweeteners, I've grown to love all-natural, organic plain yogurt with a spoonful of dark honey in it and chunks of fresh fruit. Drizzling dark honey on cheese? It is a super way to get calcium and extra antioxidants with panache.

HONEY RULE #6: Eat lean protein. I include fish (such as wild salmon and water-packed tuna) and poultry (chicken and turkey) and a few eggs per week (organic brown ones), including those used in cooking and baking. **Bit o' Honey:** I love citrus-flavored honeys on fish and poultry.

HONEY RULE #7: Savor natural desserts. I lean toward fresh fruit as my daily dessert and limit sweets (usually honey) or saturated fat to no more than a few times per week. **Bit o' Honey:** Eating honeys (no more than 100 calories per day) is okay, but I avoid eating sweets every day. Consuming a bit of honey helps to conquer cravings for the sweet treats, including ice cream, pastries, and cookies.

HONEY RULE #8: Avoid red meat. The truth is, I haven't touched meat for more than 30 years. The Mediterranean diet allows lean meat a few times per month—but I prefer not to go there. **Bit o' Honey:** Refer to honey rule #6 and try honey glazes on lean meat dishes with extra vegetables.

HONEY RULE #9: Enjoy regular exercise. I swim and walk my dogs to keep my weight and blood pressure in check, stay fit, and feel energized. **Bit o' Honey:** Eating a dark chocolate honey truffle or spoonful of creamed honey before getting physical (for extra energy) and sipping a cup of tea with honey after (to maximize the feel-good endorphins) works a workout.

HONEY RULE #10: Drink wine. If I drank, heart-healthy red wine with its antioxidants would be my choice of spirit and I would opt for moderate consumption—with meals. (I know alcohol should be avoided during pregnancy—but like an infertile worker honey bee I don't have to worry about that.) **Bit o' Honey:** I'm curious to try honey mead, but I'll save it for my next life when I get married and go on a honeymoon.

HONEY! THERE'S A NEW COMPOUND

The buzz at Oldways is that while we always knew olive oil, honey, and walnuts were good foods, new antioxidants have been found in this mighty trio, foods that are included in the Mediterranean diet. And these three foods continue to be praised. Oldways has acknowledged that these foods have been studied at the University of Granada and it's been discovered even more healthy antioxidants in phenolic compounds are in honey, oil, and walnuts. The two new techniques capillary electrophoresis and high-resolution liquid chromatography allow researchers to find these beneficial components in any plant food.

Scientists believe that these three functional foods and a medicinal herb called *Teucrium polium* are able to provide different health benefits. Findings published in the *Journal of Agricultural and Food Chemistry* show that this compound with high antioxidant activity can lower the risk of developing disease, including diabetes, cancer, heart diseases, and hypertension.[2]

Oldways says: "While these new techniques may allow us to isolate some theoretical magic bullet component in foods, we think the take-away message is a humbling one, reminding us of how little we know of what is in any food, and why it's good for us. Eating a wide variety of whole foods, especially plants, is the best way to cover our bases."

BUZZING ABOUT MEDITERRANEAN GRUB AND HONEY

What's more, honey is used as a sweetener in the Mediterranean diet. Oldways adds: "While we think it is a highly recommended sweetener, we are not sure if we can go as far as to say it is the sweetener, because other sweeteners are used as well." And that statement makes sense to me; as a dedicated follower of the Mediterranean diet, sometimes I will combine honey with raw organic sugars or even table sugar, especially in baking—all in moderation.

It's not just Oldways and me that tout this diet full of traditional Greek foods—and honey. In *The Jungle Effect: A Doctor Discovers the Healthiest Diets from Around the World—Why They Work and How to Bring Them Home* (New York: Harper Collins, 2008) author Daphne Miller, M.D., give a thumbs-up to the Mediterranean diet, too. "One study looked at Anglo Celt Australians living in Melbourne. Anglo Celts who chose to switch to a Greek-style Mediterranean diet had lower rates of diseases and lived longer than those who ate the typical Australian diet high in meat," notes the doctor, who includes 23 references to honey in *The Jungle Effect*—and includes the liquid gold in her recipes.[3]

On the topic of recipes and the Mediterranean diet, I made it a point in choosing recipes for this book that use a variety of the following common foods.

Most important, eating a variety of common Mediterranean foods and getting daily physical activity are part of the sweet package that works to lower your risk of developing diseases and ups your odds of living a longer quality life whether you reside in Europe or America. And yes, honey, olive oil, and nuts along with other common Mediterranean foods are often paired with honey, as in this honey-delicious recipe.

Common Foods and Flavors of the Mediterranean Diet Pyramid

Vegetables & Tubers	Artichokes, Arugula, Beets, Broccoli, Brussels Sprouts, Cabbage, Carrots, Celery, Celeriac, Chicory, Collard Cucumber, Dandelion Greens, Eggplant, Fennel, Kale, Leeks, Lettuce, Mache, Mushrooms, Mustard Greens, Nettles, Okra, Onions (red, sweet, white), Peas, Peppers, Potatoes, Pumpkin, Purslane, Radishes, Rutabega, Scallions, Shallots, Spinach, Sweet Potatoes, Turnips, Zucchini
Fruits	Avocados, Apples, Apricots, Cherries, Clementines, Dates, Figs, Grapefruit, Grapes, Lemons, Oranges, Melons, Nectarines, Olives, Peaches, Pears, Pomegranates, Strawberries, Tangerines, Tomatoes
Grains	Breads, Barley, Buckwheat, Bulgur, Couscous, Durum, Farro, Millet, Oats, Polenta, Rice, Wheatberries
Fish & Seafood	Abalone, Cockles, Clams, Crab, Eel, Flounder, Lobster, Mackerel, Mussels, Octopus, Oysters, Salmon, Sardines, Sea Bass, Shrimp, Squid, Tilapia, Tuna, Whelk, Yellowtail
Poultry, Eggs, Cheese, & Yogurt	Chicken, Duck, Guinea Fowl Eggs (Chicken, Quail, and Duck) Cheeses (Examples Include: Brie, Chevre, Corvo, Feta, Haloumi, Manchego, Parmigiano-Reggiano, Pecorino, Ricotta) Yogurt, Greek Yogurt
Nuts, Seeds, & Legumes	Almonds, Beans (Cannellini, Chickpeas, Fava, Kidney, Green), Cashews, Hazelnuts, Lentils, Pine Nuts, Pistachios, Sesame Seeds (Tahini), Split Peas, Walnuts
Herbs & Spices	Anise, Basil, Bay Leaf, Chiles, Clove, Cumin, Fennel, Garlic, Lavender, Marjoram, Mint, Oregano, Parsley, Pepper, Pul Biber, Rosemary, Sage, Savory, Sumac, Tarragon, Thyme, Za'atar
Meats & Sweets	Pork, Beef, Lamb, Mutton, Goat Sweets (Examples include: Baklava, Biscotti, Crème Caramel, Chocolate, Gelato, Fruit Tarts, Kunefe, Lokum, Mousse Au Chocolat, Sorbet, Tiramisu)
Water & Wine	Drink Plenty of Water Wine in Moderation

www.oldwayspt.org

Mediterranean Wrap

❖ ❖ ❖

1 cup uncooked
  couscous
½ cup chopped
  almonds, toasted
½ cup raisins
3 cups cooked,
  shredded pork
  roast
2 cups shredded
  lettuce
¼ cup honey
¼ cup olive oil
¼ cup lemon juice

2 tablespoons
  chopped fresh
  parsley
1 teaspoon curry
  powder
1 teaspoon grated
  lemon peel
Salt and pepper,
  to taste
4 pita bread pockets,
  split into 8 rounds
1 cup hummus

Cook couscous according to package directions. In medium bowl, gently combine couscous, almonds, raisins, pork, and lettuce. In small bowl, whisk together honey, olive oil, lemon juice, parsley, curry powder and lemon peel. Season with salt and pepper. Mix ¼ cup dressing into couscous mixture. To assemble wraps, lay pita rounds split side up on work surface. Spread each with 2 tablespoons hummus. Spoon approximately ½ cup couscous mixture down center of each pita round. Drizzle with 1 tablespoon dressing and fold in sides to wrap.

To Prepare Pork for Your Favorite Wrap:
Season 1½ lb. boneless pork roast with salt and pepper; brown on all sides in a hot non-stick skillet with a little olive oil. Add ½ cup chicken broth or water to pan, lower heat, cover tightly and simmer for 1 ½ hours, until roast is very tender. Check pan occasionally for liquid level; if broth has evaporated, add a little more to pan to maintain a moist cooking environment. Remove roast from pan, let cool slightly and shred or chop pork coarsely. A 1½ pound roast will yield 4 cups of pork. Use immediately or cover and refrigerate up to 4 days, until ready to use. Serve cold or reheated. Makes 4 wraps.

(*Courtesy:* National Honey Board.)

While good honey is good for you, imagine how much better it can be if it's from different honey varietals, such as alfalfa, buckwheat, and leatherwood—which have both medicinal properties and a distinct flavor. Take a look at part 3: "Honey Flavors" to see the wide, wide world of honeys and you, like me, can enjoy honeyed foods to nourish your body, mind, and spirit without taking a vacation.

UN-BEE-LIEVABLE HEALING HINTS TO CATCH

✔ On the road, purchasing honey and Mediterranean common foods was a challenge due to cash flow, but when I had them I cherished the eats like gold.

✓ ... And the Mediterranean diet includes honey, which is a recommended sweetener in the Old-ways traditional Mediterranean diet and lifestyle.

✓ The Mediterranean diet is widespread around the world and you can enjoy it wherever you are—including regular exercise.

PART 3

HONEY
FLAVORS

Healing Honey Varieties

The pedigree of Honey does not concern the Bee.
A Clover, any time, to him, Is Aristocracy.
                    —Emily Dickinson[1]

During my travels from state to state like a roving honey bee in search of a safe haven, I ended up in Eugene, Oregon. I recall one evening in the company of a nature-oriented couple who lived in a cozy house for two. The woman was an inspiration to me: Her indoor garden with a plant light, two kittens, music, and memorable tea collection amazed me. Her knowledge of each tea and how it was healing left me in awe. It was like a foreign language introduced to me that I had to learn.

When I tasted a cup of sage tea with its slightly medicinal flavor, honey came to my rescue. I knew that night that I aspired to have what she did: an all-natural, eco-friendly home amid nature and a pantry full of nature's finest, from teas to other superfoods. I craved to have the medicinal teas and honey varietals, like she did, so I could feast on them like a queen bee contented in her hive.

Still not at peace and feeling alone, I packed up my knapsack and headed north to Portland, Oregon. I found a studio apartment. I took a waitress job—swing and graveyard shifts and often back to back, like a honey bee working double shifts.

It was a sweet experience to have my own place in Portland. During the rainy days I'd bake bread and fruitcakes with a hint of honey. At night I'd serve food to the night owls. On my breaks I'd sip black tea with honey to help get through the shift—busy at midnight till 2:00 A.M., and then through the lull until breakfast full of fresh food, such as waffles and pancakes, that could have been paired with honey. The fact was, I was a human honey bee working 24 / 7 and preparing to find a new comfort zone.

Honey bees work around the nation—at home or on the road like I was doing. The warm climate of some states and of countries south of the equator allows honey bees to do their magic nearly year-round, while in colder regions the workers must cozy up in their hives during wintertime. The aroma, flavor, and color of a particular honey type are all about the type of flower from which the bee collects the nectar. Some honey shows traits of the herb or tree whose flower the bee has visited.

HONEY FLAVORS

Here, take a look at *30* popular honey varietals that I've tasted and enjoyed (thanks to dozens of honey companies). Keep in mind, polyfloral honey is made from more than one type of flower. Monofloral honey is made from one specific type—like single-origin dark chocolate—and is in demand by both beekeepers and other consumers.

There are more than 300 unique types of honey available in the United States, each coming from a different floral source. The rule is, the flavor of lighter-color honeys is milder and the flavor of darker-colored honeys is stronger. Beekeepers and people in the honey industry will also tell you that honeys with the most powerful antioxidant properties are believed to be Illinois buckwheat, California sunflower, and Hawaii Christmas berry—the dark-colored honeys that have a stronger flavor. Still, I admit that the lighter honeys are easy on the palate and the darker honeys are an acquired taste, much like dark chocolate.

These days, the flavor classifications are as follows: pleasant flavor (one that appeals to most people), acceptable flavor (one that is acceptable, though not universally appealing), unpleasant flavor (one that is acceptable to most people although not everyone's fancy), and offensive flavor (one that is not palatable by any human).[2]

Aroma of honey is a lot like flavor and these two characteristics are something to write home about for honey lovers—occasional and everyday users. The aroma of honey is described by honey authors to beekeepers by three simple words: "strong," "mild," and "weak." And personally, I love mild honeys, such as a delicate wildflower, but I am also getting used to strong honeys like buckwheat.[3]

ACACIA (*Robinia pseudoacacia*): Acacia honey (which sits in a beautiful fluted bottle in my pantry) is produced around the world, including the United States and New Zealand. Russian folk healers put acacia honey to work to treat headaches, heart disease, insomnia, kidney diseases, and respiratory ailments. *Best Blends:* Pour over fresh peaches, dates, and nuts. *My Personal Tasting:* I drizzled acacia honey over Greek honey yogurt, fresh chopped figs, and sliced almonds. This combination surpasses preflavored yogurts with a cat tail's list of artificial ingredients and sweeteners that need a translator.

ALFALFA (*Medicago sativa*): My first up-close encounter with this mild, sweet honey was when I had some fresh from the hive and put in a nice-sized jar for me. It was a gift from a local Reno, Nevada, beekeeper. The nectar source is a legume with blue flowers, and alfalfa is noted as the most popular honey in Idaho, Nevada, Oregon, Utah, and the rest of the West. It is known as a versatile honey, and its proponents claim it is used to stave off allergies. *Best Blends:* Paired with cheeses and as a good source for dressings and sauces. It is also used in tea and is a perfect table honey. *My Personal Tasting:* I used this common honey on a slice of local garlic whole-grain bread from Truckee, California. It has a slightly spicy flavor, a sierra, earthy delight. It is a good feeling to eat fresh, local food.

AVOCADO (*Persea americana*): Another western honey I befriended is found on California's avocado trees, in avocado blossoms. It's a good source of vitamins and minerals. *Best Blends:* This dark-colored honey boasts a buttery taste that works well with cheeses, dressings, and dips and premium ice cream—such as dark chocolate. *My Personal Tasting:* I bravely tried this honey on whole-wheat pancakes topped with chopped walnuts. During the hot summer months, I made a cool Greek yogurt dip with this honey for raw cruciferous vegetables.

BASSWOOD (*Tilia americana*): Not a western delight but another American honey found from Alabama to Texas and southern Canada. Basswood honey, coming from the basswood tree, is also called lime and linden honey, with a white amber color. It's a warm honey with a spicy kick. *Best Blends:* Cheese, fruit, honey mustards. *My Personal Tasting:* My first taste of basswood was stirred in plain yogurt. It was the first unopened honey jar I grabbed out of the pantry, and it won't be the last time I use this earthy delight. It reminds me of autumn—warm and savory. I also tried all-natural wheat crackers spread with goat cheese with a bit of honey on top—a superhealthful snack on a cool, crisp fall day with a crackling fire and a film on TV.

BLACKBERRY (*Rubus fruticosus*): Produced in the United States, blackberry honey has a rich berry flavor with notes of blackberry that remind me of the berries I once picked. The nectar source is wild blackberries that are found in the northwestern Pacific states—Oregon and Washington. *Best Blends:* Fruit, yogurt. *My Personal Tasting:* I enjoyed this fruity honey mixed in a bowl of granola with milk as well as on a blackberry shortcake made with whole-wheat biscuits and fresh blackberries.

BLACK LOCUST (*Robinia pseudoacacia*): Sweeter and lighter than basswood honey, this mild and pure honey is a pleasant surprise. It boasts a high fructose content. The black locust is found in North America, but its sensitivity to cold weather, and blooming in the early spring, allow locust honey to only be available sporadically in the Midwest. *Best Blends:* Paired with coffee, tea, toast, and scones. *My Personal Tasting:* I put a teaspoon in plain yogurt and fruit and was smiling because the name led me to believe it would have a strong flavor. It's a close cousin to light clover honey.

BLUEBERRY (*Vaccinium spp*): Like blackberry honey, this is another American honey with fruity notes, which comes from the blueberry bush with its tiny white flowers. It is found in the Northeast—New England—and Michigan. The honey bee is integral to blueberry plants for pollination. Blueberries and blueberry honey are rich in antioxidants. *Best Blends:* Put in teas or pour on cheese and fresh berries. *My Personal Tasting:* Just 1 teaspoon of blueberry honey made my cup of hot chamomile tea with a slice of lemon sweet and sassy. And blueberry honey is perfect with homemade blueberry–chocolate chip scones. You get a double dose of antioxidants if you use 60 percent or higher cocoa content dark chocolate. The chocolaty texture in a warmed-up scone is delicious.

BUCKWHEAT (*Fagopyrum esculentum*): Like the Golden State avocado honey, this dark delight is also grown in California and north in Washington State as well as Minnesota, Virginia, Wisconsin, and eastern Canada—but its roots are Asian. Buckwheat honey (its nectar source is the buckwheat plant) boasts more antioxidant power than the others I've noted—and contains iron. It has been touted as one of the most useful healing honeys. Buckwheat has a history with Russian folk healers of being a honey of choice, like acacia and clover honeys. Some of its healing powers include use in treating fevers, high blood pressure, and rheumatism. *Best Blends:* It is used in barbeque sauces and savory baked goods such as gingerbread and ginger snaps or as a syrup for

French toast and pancakes. *My Personal Tasting:* I opened up the jar with great curiosity, like lifting the top of Pandora's box. Too timid to try the rich honey, I put it back in the pantry to open up on another day (like in the fall when I bake a batch of chewy molasses cookies with crackled tops sprinkled with raw organic sugar).

CLOVER (*Trifolium repens*): Welcome to the most common nectar-producing plant of all honeys—familiar to most people, unlike basswood or avocado honey. Clover is the honey on the kitchen table for tea or toast. There is a variety of clover honey, with its nectar coming from red, white, alsike, and the white and yellow sweet clover plants. As with acacia honey, Russian folk healers turn to this honey, to treat atherosclerosis and to lower high blood pressure. It can also be used externally on wounds and cuts. *Best Blends:* A hint of this honey can be paired with all foods from glazes to teas, because it's a friendly and mild honey like the daisy flower. *My Personal Tasting:* I had no qualms with this all-too-familiar all-purpose honey with a mild, sweet flavor. Without hesitation I put a teaspoon in a cup of homemade lemonade and it was perfect without surprises or diving into the unknown. Clover honey is like a bite of a dark milk chocolate truffle or bar. It's the friendly honey. It's a friendly honey like a daisy is a friendly flower—one that is simple and perfect for every occasion.

CRANBERRY (*Vaccinium macrocarpon*): This fruity honey is a more exotic honey than common clover honey. Its pleasant, tart, fruity honey nectar stems from cranberry bogs, found from Wisconsin to Oregon. It boasts immune-boosting vitamin C. *Best Blends:* It is a super-match with Thanksgiving, Christmas, Valentine's Day, and other holiday dishes, including scones, poultry, and breads. *My Personal Tasting:* I tried a cranberry honey jelly that was delectable by the spoonful and on homemade muffins, from corn bread to bran.

EUCALYPTUS (*Eucalyptus spp*): From a plant grown in the Northeast, this honey is nothing like the cranberry varietal that I favor, especially in colder months. Eucalyptus has a medicinal scent, much like the essential oil or leaves. The nectar source is a tree with fragrant flowers. *Best Blends:* Pair with citrusy salad dressings and glazes for poultry. *My Personal Tasting:* This is one honey I have not tried, but I'd be most apt to team it with lemon and use it with a baked chicken breast.

FIREWEED (*Epilobium angustifolium*): Because of its name, I assumed fireweed honey would have a strong flavor, but I was pleasantly surprised. This honey comes from a perennial herb and is found in Canada and the Pacific Northwest of the United States. Somewhat like basswood, fireweed honey is light in color, "water white," and boasts a fruity, spicy, and sweet flavor. *Best Blends:* Mix with tart berries or spread on plain cakes. *My Personal Tasting:* Hungry after an afternoon swim, I grabbed a container of fireweed honey and teamed it with all-natural peanut butter on a piece of whole-grain bread. It wasn't too sweet and it sweetened my day.

GOLDENROD (*Solidago rigida*): Like clover honey, here is another versatile gem. It comes from the United States and its nectar source is a perennial with golden flowers. It's an amber color with a flowery flavor. This is one honey that attracts people with allergies. *Best Blends:* Goldenrod is a versatile honey and can enhance sweet or savory nut breads (banana to zucchini) and cheeses. *My Personal Tasting:* As a scone lover, I have baked dropped, circle, and triangle-shaped scones with every nut and fruit imaginable. I paired goldenrod honey with apple walnut scones and it gave the scones a spicy kick.

HAWAIIAN CHRISTMAS BERRY (*Schinus terebinthifolius*): Hail to another antioxidant-rich honey that is one to write home about. A healthful dark-colored honey that is derived from the Christmas berry shrub with roots in Brazil and found in Hawaii. Research at the University of Illinois showed that this honey boasts antioxidants like buckwheat honey. *Best Blends:* It is a nice addition to rich cookies and cakes. *My Personal Tasting:* Its strong flavor was best put to use by adding this honey to a batch of homemade molasses cookies sprinkled with organic sugar.

Honeydew Honey

Blossom honey or nectar honey comes from flowers and other plants and is the most popular honey. Honeydew honey, which I received from ChefShop.com, was a quality honey that I tried in plain yogurt. It is a bit different—and an exotic experience. The primary source of honeydew honey is evergreen trees in Europe. On the oval jar a honey tag penned by Giuseppe Cagnoni reads: "Honeydew Honey from organic farming; ITALIA. Honeydew honey is beautiful dark brown, free running honey and bittersweet. Bees harvest sugary secretions from the leaves of trees and convert it to honey." It takes the sophisticated palate of a devout honey lover to love honeydew honey. Organic honeydew honey is not as sweet as I thought it would be. Its rich dark color was also a surprise. Giuseppe has been creating and finding some of the finest Italian artisan honeys.

LEATHERWOOD (*Eucryphia lucida*): If you're looking for a mild honey, this exotic type derived from white-flowered leatherwood trees may not be your teaspoon of honey. This honey of Tasmania, Australia, is well known among honey lovers with a sophisticated palate—and it is an acquired taste, like 70 percent dark chocolate. A darker amber color offers decadent notes of sugar and spice. *Best Blends:* A good pair with French bread and cheeses with a strong flavor. *My Personal Tasting:* I dripped a small amount of the dark syrup over fresh, warm whole-grain French bread from the Sierra Mountains at Lake Tahoe with a few slices of sharp cheddar cheese.

LEHUA (*Metrosideros polymorpha*): If fruity honeys, such as blueberry, are your choice of sweetness, try a taste of this Hawaiian honey with an exotic twist. Called ohia, the lehua blossom tree is found in the forests on the Big Island of Hawaii. Hawaiian organic ohia lehua blossom honey is made from the blossom of the native ohia tree. Light amber in color, this honey boasts a sweet butter-scotch flavor. *Best Blends:* This Hawaiian honey is perfect with fresh fruit, premium ice creams, and homemade custard. Pairing it with fresh fruit or putting a bit in coffee will take you to the Big Island. Food in the tropics includes fish, fresh vegetables and fruits, nuts, and coffee. This honey is rare and is prized by connoisseurs for its light, delicate flavor and creamy texture. *My Personal*

Tasting: This tropical-style (my jar is from ChefShop. com) honey welcomed me on a prefall day and was a splendid and romantic surprise. I poured it over dark chocolate ice cream topped with chopped macadamia nuts. Savoring the sweet, light taste brought me, as one who has visited the Big Island several times, back to paradise.

LEMON (*Citrus limon*): Citrus lovers will love lemon blossom honey. Native to India and China, this tree grows in Italy and the United States, including California, Florida, and Texas. *Best Blends:* Lemon honey goes well with salads, poultry, glazes, teas, and desserts. *My Personal Tasting:* Creamed lemon honey is nice paired with whole-grain toast and superb with chamomile tea, and lemon honey jelly made my homemade apple scones nicer.

Manuka: The Healing Honey

Enter the superstar manuka honey (*Leptospermum scoparium*), which comes from the manuka bush. This buzzed-about New Zealand healing honey boasts a distinct flavor paired with a dark, rich amber color and gooey thick molasses texture. It's a popular honey in medical research because it does have a remarkable track record of showing super antibacterial healing properties in scientific research.

Not only does honey contain hydrogen peroxide, which has both antibacterial and antifungal properties, but it also contains a phytochemical that makes it even more extraordinary. Researchers have said it beats antibiotic-resistant strains of bacteria, such as superbug MRSA (methicillin-resistant Staphylococcus aureus).

But note, manuka honey sold as an edible honey and labeled "10+" will have the same antibacterial properties as a 10 percent phenol solution. Medical manuka honey, which should only be used topically, can go up to 20+.[4]

Research has shown that manuka honey has a high antibacterial potency, which in turn helps treat skin infections and aids digestion. It also may help to stave off gum disease. When consumed regularly (it's an acquired taste and easier to use topically) it is believed to enhance well-being.

ORANGE BLOSSOM (*Citrus sinensis*): Like other Californian honeys, this citrus favorite of mine is Asian born, but groves also are found in Arizona, Florida, and Texas. Its nectar comes from a variety of citrus sources, including orange, grapefruit, lime, and lemon trees. *Best Blends:* Goat cheese and pine nuts. Orange blossom is ideal in poultry glazes, sauces, teas, and spa beauty treatments. *My Personal Tasting:* This citrus honey, one of my favorites, gave a homemade fruit smoothie a nice tropical kick combined with fresh pineapple and coconut.

Sugar Pie, Honey Bunch

One prefall afternoon, after walking my orange and white Brittanys and in between working on this honey book, ordering wood (I was sensing it's going to be a cold fall and winter), preparing my October "Earth Changes" magazine column, I whipped up a honey peach pie. I made this Deep South sweet old-fashioned dish with an edgy twist—honey and white peaches—in the presence of my two fun-loving canines, the double-trouble sweet dog duo, who simply love it when Mom's cooking.

This time around in the kitchen, Seth, my brainiac four-year-old, put his dainty orange and white paws on the countertop and like a crafty coyote almost snagged the pie in progress. "Drop it!" I said in my best calm, assertive Dog Whisperer's type voice. My canine responded to my command on cue. The uncooked sliced peaches and pie dough didn't plop on the floor like a minor earthquake. Sethie looked up at me with his dark honey-colored eyes and said in dog-ese: *Whew! That was a close one.* The pie survived a potential pie shake-up.

I tried my hands at a lattice crust because it's different—a challenge. Peach pie is very low in cholesterol and has some protein, iron, calcium, and vitamins A and C—and fresh fruit pies are much lower in calories than cream pies. What's more, replacing refined table sugar—the white stuff—with a bit of honey will lower the high sugar content in pies. Plus, orange blossom honey is an all-purpose sweet and mild honey with a slight citrusy flavor—a fine choice for pies. The best part is twofold: the aroma of spices and honey and the perfect look fit to serve a group of queen bees.

Honey Peach Pie

❖ ❖ ❖

7–8 fresh white peaches, peeled and sliced in small wedges
1 tablespoon fresh lemon juice
½ cup white sugar
1 teaspoon of nutmeg
¼ cup of orange blossom honey
1–2 teaspoons of ground cinnamon
⅓ cup whole-wheat flour
2 tablespoons Mediterranean-style butter
2 store-bought crusts

Place peaches in a bowl. Drizzle with lemon juice. In another bowl, combine sugar, nutmeg, honey, cinnamon, and flour. Mix with fruit and add small pieces of butter. Place in one piecrust; place the other piecrust on a plate, cut into 1-inch-wide strips. Make lattice crust, placing horizontal strips first, then vertical. Flute edges. Bake pie in 350°F oven for about 50 minutes, till peaches are tender and bubbly and crust is golden brown. Cool. Serves 8.

PUMPKIN BLOSSOM (*Cucurbita pepo*): Like orange blossom, this is a favorite honey of mine, especially in autumn. Produced in Oregon and California, pumpkin blossom honey is a medium amber with a warm flavor. The nectar source is the pollination of seed crops. *Best*

Blends: Squash recipes. *My Personal Tasting:* I used this honey in homemade chocolate-chip pumpkin scones and muffins.

SAGE (*Salvia mellifera*): Welcome to a light-colored honey made from a variety of sage plants growing on the California coast and in the Sierra Nevada Mountains, like alfalfa, and near my home at Lake Tahoe. It's touted for its mild, delicate flavor. There are several varieties, including black button, white, purple, and mixed. *Best Blends:* Strong Italian cheeses, herbal teas, and fresh lemonade. *My Personal Tasting:* Sage honey brushed on a chicken breast gave it an herbal flavor and was a nice earthy change for me from using orange blossom or clover honey.

Sidr, the Priceless Honey

Meet sidr; like balsamic vinegar, this honey is pricey (it may run more than $200 a pound). A honey prized around the globe, it's guarded by Yemen's beekeepers, who go beyond the call of duty to keep it pure. Its botanical name is *Ziziphus spina-christi* and it has been tagged as sidr as well as jujube. The honey color is dark amber; the flavor is rich, and the texture is thick. Unlike other honeys that pair well with foods, this priceless gem is touted for its healing powers due to its antioxidants. Some of the health rewards you can reap from sidr include healing eye diseases, digestive woes, and respiratory infections, and it may help irregularity.

SOURWOOD (*Oxydendrum arboreum*): Ignore its name (like firewood honey) because this sweet, spicy honey is anything but sour. Its nectar source is the sourwood tree found in the Deep South, including Georgia and Alabama. This honey is noted for its versatile uses, from the table to cooking. *Best Blends:* Sweet berry bagels, green tea, glazed poultry. *My Personal Tasting:* I spread a homemade whole-wheat biscuit with sourwood honey and paired it with a veggie omelet and the combo was perfect, not too sweet and not too spicy, with a southern fix.

STAR THISTLE (*Centaurea solstitialis*): Another versatile table honey like clover is star thistle. Touted as a noteworthy weed and plant, star thistle is found in the Midwest, California, and Oregon. It has a good flavor with a spicy punch to it. *Best Blends:* A nice sweetness to drip on nuts and cheeses. *My Personal Tasting:* Star thistle spread on warm homemade corn bread makes for a delicious comfort food as a snack or paired with a bowl of hearty soup.

SUNFLOWER (*Helianthus annuus*): Another impressive honey that wowed me is sunflower, probably because it boasts an Italian flair. In my living room above the fireplace mantel is artwork of sunflowers—the nectar source is the flower head. This honey is from sunflowers found in Georgia and the northern United States, including North and South Dakota. *Best Blends:* Good with fresh fruit, savory breads, and Greek yogurt. *My Personal Tasting:* My first taste of thick and creamy Greek yogurt included sunflower honey and slices of juicy purple grapes. It was a memorable Tuscany-type treat without having to leave Northern California and one I probably would find easily south in Napa, wine country.

TULIP POPLAR (*Liriodendron tulipifera*): This versatile honey, like clover but a bit stronger, is also a southern favorite. On tall trees with large greenish-yellow flowers from the Gulf States to New England and south Michigan honey bees will be found. The color of this honey is dark amber, but the flavor is milder than you'd expect from a dark honey. It's rich and sweet. *Best Blends:* A teaspoon or two on top of all-natural French vanilla ice cream; spread on pancakes and muffins; used in gingerbread and molasses cookies. *My Personal Tasting:* I spread this honey on homemade corn-bread muffins and used it in a batch of bran muffins.

TUPELO (*Nyssa ogeche*): A premium honey thanks to tupelo trees found in Florida and southern Georgia. Tupelo honey is light amber in color, with a greenish hue. Tupelo honey boasts a mild, notable taste. Due to its high fructose content it will not crystallize for a long time. *Best Blends:* A nice honey topped over blue and robust cheeses; a glaze for pork. *My Personal Tasting:* I have not tried this honey yet due to the fact that it is in a beautiful tapered bottle and is so pretty to look at it is difficult to open the bottle and pair the honey with edibles.

WHITE HONEY (*Prosopis pallida*): If you get a chance to give your taste buds a rare treat, open your eyes and heart to a rare Hawaiian organic honey. It comes from the flowers of the Kiawe tree. This tree grows at sea level in nearby desert regions on the leeward side of the Big Island of Hawaii. It is a single floral source of certified organic, unheated raw honey. *Best Blends:* This exotic honey can be tossed with fresh seasonal fruit, salty, strong-flavored, and even stinky cheeses, and coffee or tea. *My Personal Tasting:* Vosges Haut-Chocolat combines efforts with Richard Spiegel's Volcano Island Honey

Company. This seasonal gourmet chocolate company uses the white honey on one side next to a dark ganache, forming a decadent truffle. Each truffle is one-half organic white honey, one-half dark chocolate ganache. It is also sweet right off the spoon, which I've tried before swimming.

WILDFLOWER: This well-loved honey by honey fans and *moi* is found around the world in an infinite number of flowers. It can be a mild, rich honey from a combination of spring, summer, and fall flowers. Autumn wildflower comes from fall plants like goldenrod, so this honey is dark, strong flavored, and rich in antioxidants. *Best Blends:* Regular wildflower honey works well in teas and drizzled over tea cakes and fresh seasonal fruit. Autumn wildflower is best in baking and sauces. *My Personal Tasting:* I simply adore regular wildflower—it's a perfect honey at Lake Tahoe, touted for its wildflowers that bloom in late spring and summertime—and have used it on homemade strawberry shortcake.

Rare Hawaiian Smoothie

❖ ❖ ❖

1 medium papaya
2 small bananas
¼ cup apple juice
¼ cup orange juice
2 tablespoons Rare Hawaiian Organic White Honey
1 tablespoon peanut butter
1 tablespoon nutritional yeast
2 teaspoons lemon juice
1 pinch of sea salt
6 ice cubes

Blend all ingredients until smooth. Delight yourself and your friends with approximately three 8-ounce servings of this delicious, nutritious Rare Hawaiian Smoothie!

(*Source:* Volcano Island Honey Company.)

HONEY CRÈMES

Creamed honey is a form of the nectar of the gods that you'll fancy because of its texture and delectable taste. Honey crèmes are blended with fruits or spices. A super bonus: These gems stay smooth without refrigeration and can be savored by the spoonful or paired with a variety of edibles. Here's just a taste of what you can get from the hive.

Honey Crème	Flavor	Uses
Apricot Crème	Notes of apricot	Toast, scones, muffins, pancakes, waffles, coffees, and teas
Blackberry Crème	Blackberries mixed in pure honey	Biscuits, bagels, and hot beverages
Clover Crème	All-natural honey	French toast, breads, muffins, and scones
Cranberry Crème	Sweet-tart cranberries	Tea breads, muffins, biscuits, and oatmeal

| Raspberry Crème | Raspberries mixed in pure honey | Topping for waffles and pound cake |
| Spiced Crème | Pure whipped honey with cinnamon and other spices | Mixed with cream cheese for a topping for bagels and as a dip for apples and gingerbreads |

(*Source:* Honey Ridge Farms.)

Mix It Up

Flavored/fruited honey is honey that has fruit, coloring, or flavoring added. Infused honey is a honey that has had flavors of herbs, peels, and spices added to it by steeping. Mix-Ins is another honey mixture that surprised me, thanks to Helene Marshall of Marshall's Farm Honey. We're talking Honey & Apples, Honey & Almonds, Honey & Walnut Halves. "I produce the Mix-Ins because they are so wonderful to taste, and use with other dishes. All we do is mix honey and nuts and / or fruits together," she told me. And I discovered another honey delight.

If you pair the nut honeys with Greek yogurt, like I did, you've got a healthful and sophisticated treat. Nut honeys are a gourmet wonder. "The almonds soak up the sweet nectar of the honey and the honey absorbs naturally the nuttiness of the almond," explains Marshall, who adds that the Mix-Ins also pair nicely with breads, cheese dishes, rice, pancakes, waffles, and a host of culinary creations. And yes, I did eat the "nutted honey" right out of the jar. No refrigeration needed; since honey is a preservative, it also preserves what's in it, adds the honey guru.

Spices, including allspice, anise, cinnamon, cloves, and nutmeg, are also used to flavor honey. But it doesn't stop there. Vanilla, citrus, and ginger are part of the pack, as well as other things that are for people who love pure honeys but also love to add a little spice to their nectar.

ARTISANAL HONEY SAUCES AND DRESSINGS

Honey goes well with some ingredients that will surprise you and your palate. Artisan producers (and chefs) are combining honeys with good-for-you foods, too. Not only do the honeyed sauces and dressings add an extra exotic touch to your foods, but they also add irresistible flavor that will make you want to share the sweetness with family and friends.

BALSAMIC VINEGAR: For 1,000 years, balsamic vinegar, coined "Aceto Balsamico," has been valued for its medicinal properties. As with red wine vinegar, its grape-filled counterpart, balsamic vinegar contains powerful antioxidants that protect against heart disease—and may even fight cancer. *Best Honey Blend:* Balsamic Honey Vinegar is a honey lover's must-have product. Honey Ridge Farms sent me a bottle. Made from 100 percent honey, it's sulfite free and delicately balances sweet with tart, adding depth and flavor to a variety of recipes. The grape-based honey vinegar can be used for salad dressings, marinades, and sauces or drizzled on vanilla ice cream. A bonus: One tablespoon contains a mere 25 calories and no cholesterol, sodium, or fat. That's sweet. But there's more. . . .

Artisan honey vinegars are combinations of honey vinegar with herbs, spices, and other wholesome ingredients. These honey vinegars, from lemongrass coriander to sun-dried tomato and tarragon, pair nicely with salads, vegetables, sandwiches, sauces, and even soups. I favor the honey vinegar from Honey Ridge Farms, but you can get honey vinegar at specialty shops and other online merchants.

CHOCOLATE: Imagine an Italian chocolate sauce sweetened with honey. It is the ultimate dessert topping and a treat in coffee or for dipping chunks of fresh fruit. Ingredients are pure and simple: cocoa and honey. Thank you, Magnolia Honey Company; this Chocolate Lace sauce continues to make my day and night.

OLIVE OIL: Olive oil, like balsamic vinegar and other vinegars, has been combined for health and beauty. Combining extra virgin olive oil with honey gets you plenty of disease-fighting polyphenols—and flavor. Plus, you're using a healthful fat and choice sweetener. *Best Honey Blend:* Olive oil and honey sauces and dressings are available at your health-food store and grocery store and online. Also, recipes—cooking and baking—from breakfast dishes to entrees, often combine olive oil and honey. (See chapter 13: "Honey Bee-autiful" for honey and olive oil treatments and chapter 18: "Ciao, Honey!" for recipes.)

JUDGING A TASTE OF HONEY

When I began receiving honeys, I was a bit overwhelmed. I opened up each box, week by week, and the jars of honey increased in number to dozens. One question that was nagging me was: How the heck do I judge the taste of the different varieties?

With chocolate, I had my own judging formula. If it worked, the chocolate was gone in less than a week. The chocolate that was put into my file cabinet and collected cobwebs didn't make the cut. But honey is a different type of tasting. If I cooked or baked with each and every one, my petite size might change to give me the look of a spayed middle-aged cat. So, I went straight to the source of honey knowledge—Delicious Italy—to get the answer. Here, take a look at the six-step process:

1. Place the honey of choice in the classic balloon-shaped glass.
2. Warm the honey by cupping your hand around the glass and the light heat will release the natural scent and make the honey slightly more liquid.
3. Check for impurities by holding it to the light, then taking a spoon and allowing the honey to fall back into the glass.
4. Our taste buds recognize sweet, salt, acidic, and bitter properties. The tip of the tongue is where the sweetness of the honey will hit first.
5. A strong-flavored honey will also have a so-called *retronasale,* which will appear at the back of the nose.
6. The more soluble honeys contain more fructose, the less soluble more glucose.

Putting to work a honey varietal in a recipe is fun and the possibilities are endless and exciting when you get creative, like in the following recipe, and add tea to give it an extra kick.

Honey and Lemon Green Tea Cupcakes

❖ ❖ ❖

½ cup boiling water
1 green tea bag
2 cups unbleached all-purpose flour
½ teaspoon baking soda
½ teaspoon baking powder
½ teaspoon salt

Zest and juice (¼ cup) of one lemon
¼ cup buttermilk
½ cup butter, softened
¾ cup Orange Blossom honey
2 large eggs

Preheat oven to 350°F. Pour boiling water over tea bag and steep 3 minutes. Remove tea bag and allow tea to cool. Sift together flour, baking soda, baking powder and salt; set aside. In a liquid measure, combine green tea, lemon zest and juice, and buttermilk; set aside. In a mixing bowl, cream butter until fluffy. Add honey; mix well. Add eggs, one at a time. Add half of the reserved dry ingredients to the butter mixture; mix on low until just combined. With mixer running on low, slowly add the lemon tea mixture. Add remaining dry ingredients until just combined. Fill paper-lined muffin tins ⅔ full. Bake 18–22 minutes, or until a toothpick inserted in center of a muffin comes out clean. Remove to wire rack; cool. Frost and decorate with Honey Lemon Frosting and Candied Lemon Slices (below), if desired. Note: Any mild-flavored honey such as clover may be used. Makes 12–14 cupcakes.

CANDIED LEMON SLICES AND HONEY LEMON FROSTING

¼ cup Orange Blossom honey
1 lemon, thinly sliced
½ cup butter, softened

4 cups powdered sugar, sifted
¼ cup lemon juice
½ teaspoon lemon zest

Preheat oven to 200°F. Pour honey in a small skillet and add lemon slices in a single layer. Bring to a boil over medium heat. Reduce heat and simmer for 15 to 20 minutes, turning slices occasionally. Remove from heat; reserve syrup. Place slices on a parchment-lined cookie sheet and bake 10 minutes. Turn slices and bake an additional 10 minutes or until slices are dry. In a mixing bowl, cream butter until light and fluffy. Add 2 cups of powdered sugar; mix well. Slowly add cooled reserved syrup and lemon juice and zest; mix well. Add remaining powdered sugar; beat well. *Any mild-flavored honey such as clover may be used. Makes 12–14 servings.

(*Source:* National Honey Board.)

Now that I've infused some flavored honeys into your brain, in the next chapter you'll find out how teaming cinnamon, an ancient superspice used since biblical times, and honey is good for you, from head to toe (excluding the myths) and tastes amazing, too.

UN-BEE-LIEVABLE HEALING HINTS TO CATCH

- ✓ Honey varietals come from different shrubs, trees, flowers, and other plants—offering you different flavors and aromas.
- ✓ Polyfloral honey is made from more than one type of flower; monofloral is made from one specific type—like single-origin dark chocolate.
- ✓ The darker the honey, the more antioxidants and the stronger the flavor.
- ✓ Honeys offer different healing powers. Manuka and sidr stick out on the list of standout honeys.
- ✓ Honey, dark, light, or antioxidant richer than others, gets better when infused with nature's herbs, spices, and fruits. Not only do these ingredients boost flavor and texture—they can also add more vitamins, minerals, and antioxidants.
- ✓ Herbs, spices, and fruits can enhance your immune system, lower risk of heart disease and can-

cer, help you to lose unwanted weight, and do much more.

✓ Flavored / fruited honey and Mix-In honeys give you more flavor and healthful herbs, peels, and spices.

✓ Artisanal honey sauces and dressings paired with olive oil, vinegar, and chocolate offer extra healing powers.

PART 4

MORE HEALING SUPERFOODS

CHAPTER 8

Honey and Cinnamon Power

Cinnamon bites and kisses simultaneously.
—Vanna Bonta[1]

I faced sweet and spicy experiences on my road travels, like a honey bee in flight; I was stricken by untimely challenges. One afternoon in Las Vegas, Tiger and I were in front of Lady Luck Casino. It was my idea to leave my long-haired partner in the shade with water at the doorstep of the entryway while I tried to hitch a safe ride back home to California. As I was walking inside, an older man called out to me, "Nice dog!" I got an uneasy vibe but tuned it out.

Fifteen minutes later, I left the casino. My best friend was MIA. Shocked and disoriented like a beekeeper with stolen bee colonies, I stood outside in the hot sun. I tried to fight back the tears. After a long search there was no rescue. My canine buddy was gone. I cried all night long.

At dawn, at a café I ordered a cinnamon roll, tea, and honey. I was like a devoted beekeeper without his bees. I was alone. It was one of the worst experiences I endured on the road. And flashbacks of our travels from coast to coast haunted me then but now are cherished memories of a dog and a girl—an amazing human–animal bond. I left a photo of me, the hippie girl with her dog in Ontario, on the bulletin board at the local animal shelter. Through all the pain and loss, I moved on.

A few months later, fate paid me a visit. A black Labrador pup with soulful brown eyes came into my life on the road. We rescued each other at Ocean Beach, San Diego. We bonded instantly like a beekeeper with new queens, and Stone Fox and I, California Butterfly, continued on our journey together. A loyal dog and its dedicated human are similar to the superpowers of two superfoods—honey and cinnamon.

HONEY'S CONSTANT COMPANION

The delicious taste of hot cinnamon buns with sticky honey and the scent of homemade apple pie baking in the oven evoke memories from my childhood. The earthy, inviting flavor of cinnamon has been used worldwide by a multitude of cultures for its versatile seasoning powers as well as for its healing powers, for thousands of years.

Cinnamon comes from the bark of the cinnamon tree found mostly in Ceylon and China. It can be found in several forms, including the stick, which can be grated or used to stir or season beverages—such as hot chocolate and apple cider. In ground form, cinnamon is the most common spice used for seasoning and baking. There are countless dishes that call for both cinnamon and honey—two of nature's finest foods that complement each other as well as provide medicinal properties.

A new feature on the Mediterranean diet pyramid is the addition of spices, for reasons of both health and taste. Also, spices contribute to the natural identities of various Mediterranean cuisines.

So, can a spice, like cinnamon, paired with honey, which enhances the taste of many foods and warms the hearts of all who enjoy its aroma, hold healing powers to relieve pain and rev up your sex drive? I took a look at the popular claims and this is what I discovered.

HONEY AND CINNAMON HEALTH BENEFITS: 10 REAL REASONS THE DUO IS SWEET

Honey and cinnamon have a lot in common. Like honey, cinnamon's healing powers have been praised from folk medicine since biblical times to the modern day. Cinnamon's powers can help prevent age-related diseases and conditions such as cancer, heart disease, and obesity.

Cinnamon, like honey, contains antioxidants. Also, both functional foods are used for home cures. You'll also discover both cinnamon and honey provide natural healing powers from head to toe. Here, take a look at the real research behind the claims concerning this powerful duo.

1 **Aphrodisiac:** Is cinnamon really a way to reignite passion? Perhaps it is, according to past research at the Smell & Taste Treatment & Research Foundation in Chicago, Illinois. When men were ex-

posed to dozens of scents, the only one that got a positive sexual response was the aroma of hot cinnamon buns.

The Real Honey and Cinnamon Cure: Refer to chapter 18: "Ciao, Honey!" for cinnamon and honey recipes to get that romantic touch with cinnamon and honey. If that doesn't provide results, at least you'll be getting nature's sweetest foods with nutritional benefits—without fat or cholesterol—and that can also help enhance libido for both men and women.

2 **Arthritis:** Aches and pains from creaky cartilage and joints, like a lackluster love life, can wreak havoc on your lifestyle and well-being. While cinnamon is not a magic bullet for gaining flexibility and losing pain, it does contain anti-inflammatory compounds that may be beneficial in reducing pain and stiffness in muscles and joints.

The Real Honey and Cinnamon Cure: Try a cup of cinnamon tea teamed with a fresh cinnamon stick and a teaspoon of honey. You may get the pain relief from the anti-inflammatory compounds in cinnamon, and the honey (also with anti-inflammatory properties) will provide instant energy so you can do daily stretches (or even make love, and that'll provide relief of pain due to the feel-good endorphins).

3 **Cholesterol:** While pain isn't fun, tallying up out-of-whack cholesterol numbers is no picnic, either. Powerful phytochemicals in cinnamon can reduce blood sugar, as well as triglycerides (fat in your blood), total cholesterol, and LDL "bad" cholesterol in people with type 2 diabetes. Team

that with honey, which has no fat or cholesterol, and you may just be able to keep your cholesterol levels healthy.

The Real Honey and Cinnamon Cure: Incorporate honey and cinnamon powder in your diet regime, which should be a low-fat, low-cholesterol diet. Also, if you are overweight, honey and cinnamon can help you to lose weight to keep your "good" HDL cholesterol numbers up. Don't forget B vitamin–rich foods, such as fish with a honey glaze or a smoothie with wheat germ and honey for vitamin B_6 and French toast with egg, milk, and honey or poultry with a honey glaze for vitamin B_{12}.

4 **Colds:** If cinnamon and honey can help keep sugar levels steady, can it stave off a common cold? There are many home-cure remedies that call for honey and cinnamon to help cure the common cold. Does it work? This combo cold buster may help stave off a common cold as well as speed up your recovery due to its antibacterial and antiviral properties. But if your immune system has been compromised and you're keeping company with someone who has a cold, cinnamon and honey may not be 100 percent effective.

The Real Honey and Cinnamon Cure: Adding tea to your daily diet regime, especially antioxidant-rich green and black tea, paired with honey and cinnamon, can help you to keep your immune system strong so if you do catch a cold, you'll be able to kick the virus faster.

5 **Hair Loss:** A cinnamon-honey cure may keep you well, but can it maintain a strong mane? When I

think of cinnamon and honey as a cure-all for thinning hair, the classic *I Love Lucy* episode "Ricky Thinks He's Going Bald" comes to mind. In the kitchen she puts her husband through "guaranteed" scalp treatments. It's absurd, and believing a spice and superfood concoction is going to halt hair loss is ridiculous. Hair loss is due to many factors, including genetics, aging, stress, and a poor diet.

The Real Honey and Cinnamon Cure: If your family tree is on your side, then you may be able to stall Father Time (and hair loss) by learning to chill, and honey can help you to do just that. (See part 6: "Honey Cures.") Also, using both cinnamon and honey in your daily diet may help you keep your mane (or what's left of it) because each contains antiaging, disease-fighting antioxidants.

6 **Immune System:** Honey and cinnamon may be a useful cold buster as well as bolstering your immunity against disease from the flu to cancer. The caveat: You need to also bolster your immunity in healthful ways, from a nutrient-rich immunity-boosting diet to exercise and a healthy lifestyle (i.e., minimizing distress and getting adequate shut-eye), to keep bugs and superbugs at bay.

The Real Honey and Cinnamon Cure: Taking 1 to 2 teaspoons daily multiple times per week along with including antioxidant-rich honey and cinnamon in nutrient-rich meals can help bolster your immunity. Also, drink green tea and a teaspoon of honey (especially acacia and sunflower varieties) once or twice a day.

7 Infertility: Yes, the honey-cinnamon pair can help keep sickness at bay, but can it also help a woman to get pregnant? Ayurveda medicine practitioners tout honey for helping both genders achieve fertility wonders. However, my left side of the brain (the practical one that thinks and reasons) says you would have better luck asking a psychic advisor for a magic potion.

The Real Honey and Cinnamon Cure: But note, some men and women who are stressed out trying to conceive may be sabotaging their goal. In other words, relaxing has been said to help couples get pregnant. That said, because honey can help to calm nerves and cinnamon can help the body stay clear of diabetes and unhealthy cholesterol, the spicy-sweet cure can do more good than harm. Your best bet: Bake a batch of Cinnamon Honey Buns and let nature take its course.

8 Longevity: So, if the honey-cinnamon combo can enhance your immune system and fight diabetes, it just may add years to your life, or not. There are elderly folks, from 80 to 100 plus, who pop up from time to time in the news to remind us that they include the golden nectar in their golden years. Also, these same people are often down-to-earth people who eat nature's foods, which include herbs and spices—like cinnamon.

The Real Honey and Cinnamon Cure: Like going bald, living a long life often is linked to genes. Can we give credit to honey and cinnamon for helping humans to live to 100 years old? Again, the left brain tells me it's a mixed bag of strategies, including a healthful diet, regular exercise, social bonds, a purpose in life, and staving off unhealthy lifestyle habits, that is key to longevity—not sweet honey and spicy cinnamon. Still, if you include these two superfoods in your day-to-day life along with a wholesome lifestyle, then yes, my right brain says, *Honey and Cinnamon Power!*

9 **Stomach Upset:** From hairless to queasy—can honey and cinnamon come to the rescue if your stomach is turning topsy-turvy? The sweetener and spice are tummy friendly. Cinnamon is a carminative—which simply means it can help relieve gas. If it works for you, no doctor or rat study should work against you and convince you to turn down the honey and cinnamon home cure, because it may work for your ailment.

The Real Honey and Cinnamon Cure: A hot cup of tea, such as ginger (which is proven to soothe an upset stomach or nausea), or low-fat milk with a teaspoon of honey and cinnamon powder or a fresh stick can calm your nerves—and that may indeed help get rid of queasies.

10 **Weight Loss:** Last but not the least mind-boggling, can honey and cinnamon be the ticket to a lean body? Some folks say yes, these two superfoods can help you to shed unwanted pounds ASAP. While I do believe both honey and cinnamon can help you, if you don't exercise and do still overindulge in food, no, a "Honey and Cinnamon Miracle Diet" will not work. Still, honey can help you to cut sweet cravings, so if a sweet tooth is ruining your dieting efforts, honey can come to the rescue. Cinnamon adds flavor to foods, such as oatmeal,

so you won't be tempted to use high-fat butter or added sugars.

The Real Honey and Cinnamon Cure: Each day, try drinking 2 cups of fat-burning green tea and cinnamon powder. Not only will the tea and cinnamon help rev up your metabolism, but the honey will also help give you energy so you'll stick to physical exercise and burn more calories.

Whether you're looking to get that loving feeling or fighting a cold, eating one Cinnamon Honey Bun, like in the following recipe, paired with a cup of hot herbal tea, will make you feel good and just may help to follow through on battling your health woe and do its job. And there is always the chance that the aroma in your kitchen will rev up the romance in your life.

Cinnamon Honey Buns

❖ ❖ ❖

¼ cup butter or margarine, soft- and divided
½ cup honey, divided
½ cup chopped toasted nuts, optional

⅔ cup raisins
2 teaspoons ground cinnamon
1 pound frozen bread dough, thawed according to package directions

Grease 12 muffin cups with 1 tablespoon butter. To prepare honey nut topping, mix together 1 tablespoon butter, ¼ cup honey and chopped nuts. Place 1 teaspoon topping in each muffin cup. To prepare filling, mix together remaining 2 tablespoons butter, remaining ¼ cup honey and cinnamon. Roll out bread dough onto floured surface into 18 x 8–inch rectangle. Spread filling evenly over dough. Sprinkle evenly with raisins. Starting with long side, roll dough into log. Cut log into 12 (1½–inch) slices. Place 1 slice, cut-side up, into each prepared muffin cup. Set muffin pan in warm place; let dough rise for 30 minutes. Place muffin pan on foil-lined baking sheet. Bake at 375°F 20 minutes or until buns are golden brown. Remove from oven; cool in pan 5 minutes. Invert muffin pan to remove buns. Makes 12 buns.

(*Source:* National Honey Board.)

In the next chapter, "Sweet Stuff: Honey Combos," you'll discover that honey is found in a variety of foods, from breads and candy to ice cream and yogurt. The best part is, yes, these combinations are often good for you, thanks to healing honey and its powers.

UN-BEE-LIEVABLE HEALING HINTS TO CATCH

✓ Cinnamon and honey are both chock-full of antioxidants—which can lower the risk of heart disease and cancer and increase longevity.

✓ Pairing cinnamon and honey can give you a double dose of antioxidants and essential minerals and vitamins, too.

✓ Cinnamon and honey provide real health benefits, including revving up your sex drive, boosting your immune system, soothing an upset stomach, and helping in weight loss . . .

✓ . . . but note, cinnamon and honey cannot take credit on this planet for growing hair and making babies.

✓ Using cinnamon and honey both inside and outside of your body for total health care can be good for your mind and spirit.

Sweet Stuff: Honey Combos

If you have no honey in your Pot, have some in your Mouth.

—Benjamin Franklin[1]

After I worked hard for the money in Oregon, like a worker bee transported to pollinate crops, my devoted dog, Stone Fox, and I fled back to the Golden State. We landed in Hollywood, Southern California. It is a region full of honey bees and warm weather where I ended my journey—for a while. We were given refuge by a communal-type group of like-minded artistic, fun-loving people, much like a bee colony.

My job was kitchen duty: cooking and baking. One day before a coastal picnic, I baked a batch of chocolate-chip cookies. I didn't have a gourmet kitchen in our Bohemian-type apartment. I was resourceful. There was no table sugar in the house, so I turned to honey as my main sweetener. I remember sipping iced tea laced with honey from our favorite health-food store *and* nibbling on semi-sweet chocolate chips during the baking process from beginning to end.

Teaming the sweet pair worked like a bee charmer. The cookies were savored by my friends, much like hungry worker bees feeding on nectar. I felt like a queen bee must feel (yes, I believe honey bees have emotions like dogs and cats do), content with a good colony and reaping rewards of good sweets.

THE SWEET THINGS

Move over, sugar; honey is the up-and-coming sweet thing on the block. The use of honey in foods is becoming more popular, thanks to the health wave of the 21st century. Think dark honey instead of white sugar— like dark chocolate instead of milk chocolate—that's making a big splash worldwide.

Credit goes to consumers for demanding honey-based products, according to Global Industry Analysts. A hike in the variety and assortment of honey-based food products, such as yogurts and drinks, is because we know honey is "an appealing ingredient as compared to artificial sweeteners." What's more, honey is out of the closet and touted for its antioxidants, minerals, vitamins, and proteins, so it's getting well-deserved attention.[2]

Each time I go to the grocery store, I notice that the word "honey" is put in big print on boxes, cartons, and packages of products such as breads, breakfast cereals, candy, honey drinks, ice cream, yogurt, and much more. Countless products touting honey's all-natural, wholesome image are available to the consumer, like you and me, every day. Here, meet some sweet honey combos that are making a buzz . . .

Breads and Baking Mixes: Corn-bread mix, packaged wheat bread, and pancake and biscuit mixes are just some foods that boast that five letter word "h-o-n-e-y." One time I grabbed a honey pancake mix and was as excited as a forager bee in spring, ready to try it with fresh blueberries. My excitement plummeted when I read the label: "powdered honey." I thought, *I'd rather use a real, raw natural liquid honey to have control of my sweet honey pancakes.* And I made honey pancakes from scratch and monitored my honey addition.

Fresh-baked store-bought breads that include honey are a different species of honey foods, especially if the ingredient label lists "honey" without the word "powdered." Honey helps baked goods last long, since it's a good preservative, and that works for me.

Breakfast Cereal: As with breads and pancakes, I prefer to use liquid honey on oatmeal or granola, especially when I can control the honey type. Each bowl of cereal can be a new and exciting experience, unlike if you eat the prepackaged honey-sweetened cereals. But I've enjoyed natural honey granolas (with real honey) and Honey Nut Cheerios (with real honey).

Candy: In candies, honey is used in different countries, in such products as nougat (a confection made from a honey paste and nuts) from France and halva (a confection of crushed sesame seed in a binder of honey) from Greece. It is believed that honey may not be the sweetener of choice for caramels because its nature to quickly absorb moisture will lessen the time before the expiration date and soften the candy, which may end up as one sticky blob.

But I didn't have that problem with Vosges milk chocolate caramels with tupelo honey and bee pollen. Nor did I have a sticky mess with Lake Champlain Caramel Five Star Bar (with fresh Vermont cream, butter, sugar, honey, and vanilla, slow-cooked in copper kettles, yielding creamy caramel; dark chocolate chunks and almonds are added and covered in milk chocolate). The Chocolate's Honey Caramels are 1¼-inch-in-diameter and ½-inch-thick round candy pieces boasting a beehive and wildflowers decorating dark chocolate, filled with caramel and laced with honey. Wrapped in embossed Italian gold foil, these honey caramels are the ultimate gift for honey lovers, like me, who often have honey and chocolate on the brain.

During my search for the ultimate honey candy, I quickly learned that many honey candies, such as honey salt water taffy and gourmet honey jelly beans, use honey flavoring—not real honey. But that wasn't always the case.

I was sent a box of Manuka Honey & Rainforest Lemon Delight that delighted me and probably would do the same for a honey bee. It is a fusion of New Zealand manuka honey and Australian lemon myrtle (plus sugar, glucose, and wheat starch). The rub is, the item is imported from New Zealand and it's not cost-effective for the product to be shipped to the United States. (If you go to or live in Karori Wellington, New Zealand, check out Loukoumi, Ltd.) The lemon delight's counterpart Honey & Hazel Delight was inspired by traditional Mediterranean recipes. Loukoumi blended roasted hazelnuts with honey from New Zealand. Note to self: Relocate to down under, where I can have a constant supply of these candies.

Honey Drinks: Good-for-you honey drinks, much like healthful vinegar concoctions, are popular in Asian countries such as Japan. Honey drinks are often paired with lemon juice for a sweet and tart twist. To fruit juices, coffee, and tea honey is added as the primary and / or sole sweetener. And I prefer pure honey rather than honey-flavored syrups and artificial sweeteners with honey. It's a nature granola-girl thing. Honey is my preferred sweet thing in beverages and crunchy treats.

Honey Ice Cream: Adding honey to calcium-rich ice creams sounds like a sweet idea, right? Not so much. It is believed that honey ice creams may melt faster than those made with sugar. As a lover of Häagen-Dazs ice cream and their Vanilla Honey Bee ice cream, I didn't have a meltdown issue. Out of curiosity, though, I put two premium vanilla ice creams to the test. Yes, the honey ice cream did melt a bit faster, but this is a moot point to me because when I dish up a scoop it is meant to be eaten, not a decoration to admire.

Honey Nuts: Honey-glazed almonds, cashews, walnuts, and other nuts are easily found in grocery stores and online specialty shops, and you can make them, too. Nuts are a healthful food chock-full of monounsaturated fat and protein and play a role in the Mediterranean diet—like honey—if eaten in moderation. I tried Honey Roasted Cashews from Oh! Nuts, an online company. These honey-glazed cashews are all-natural sweet candy. The ingredients: cashews, sugar, cottonseed and / or canola oil, and honey. One serving is a mere 150 calories, with protein, iron, and calcium. The flavor was earthy, full flavored, and the sweetest thing with a crunch.

Snack Bars: Honey is thick and sticky like "bee glue," which certainly can help bind a bar—homemade or store-bought—and gives snack bars a sweet and healthful flavor. Good, crunchy honey and oats granola bars and chewy protein bars—many brands—provide a list of healthful, all-natural ingredients, and honey is one of them, which is a good thing. Speaking of health . . .

Yogurt: Honey is used as a sweetener in Greek yogurt. This is better than yogurts that have been sweetened with artificial ingredients. Honey is the real thing. I prefer to use a spoonful of my own honey in a cup of yogurt, but sometimes for convenience, if you're not at home, a honey yogurt would be a perfect thing.

A Honey of a Tale

As the story goes, in a valley at the foot of the Rocky Mountains just east of Yellowstone National Park in northern Wyoming is a small farm where Clarence and Bessie Zeller raised their family of three sons and three daughters.

To support the family, they produced honey. This honey was made by bees they called Little Johnnies. The term originated from the wild bees Clarence's father took from the bee trees on the Shoshone River bottoms. Little Johnnies are mean, and they attack just for the fun of it. They just love to sting, but they gather the sweetest nectar, which makes this special honey.

Bessie began creating the honey candy more than 50 years ago thanks to an optometrist. He pointed out to her that her son Mitchel's vision would improve if sugar was not part of his diet. In a quest for a natural sugar, she turned to honey. "One year later, he didn't need glasses," says the candy maker.

When the boys grew up, they left home. Time passed. The sting of the Little Johnnies was like the Pied Piper calling them back to the farm and their beloved bees.

In 1976, they decided to make use of an old family recipe from Bessie's ancestors in Scotland and make honey candy for sale. The boys had made taffy as kids and had lots of fun stretching it. They had all the necessary ingredients for delicious candy—that special honey, the recipe, and the desire. More recipes were developed, and in 1979 they started making honey pecan pralines, now known as Pecan Pearls. And then the chocolate and honey candies followed.

In the Queen Bee Gardens gourmet candy catalog, words tout the healing powers of both honey and chocolate. Researchers believe that chocolate's appeal, like that of honey, is a combo of its nutrients and chemical composition, as well as fat and sugar. Naturally, it's noted that "all chocolates are not created equal"—reminding you to look for chocolate containing no hydrogenated fat and oils. Chocolate is considered high quality if the only fat is cocoa butter. The best chocolate should be low in sugar. And, as with honey products, choose a chocolate with few added ingredients or fillings that are high in fat or sugar. But the stand-out honey candy doesn't stop there. . . .

Queen Bee Gardens is on top of the benefits of pollen—"the natural food with enzymes, antioxidants and vitamins." Queen Bee's Pollen Drops are unique among candies. Developed as a nutritional supplement, they not only taste great but also contain nutritious elements. Pollen Drops are made with fresh-from-the-hive honey, creamery butter, dry milk, algin, and vanilla. Stretched to give them a fine texture, Pollen Drops are a taffy. To preserve the nutrients in the pollen, it is stretched into the candy only after the candy has been cooled, giving it that golden color.

(*Source:* Queen Bee Gardens gourmet candy catalog.)

HONEY AND CHOCOLATE

Honey and chocolate are both superfoods that have been used since biblical times. The healing benefits of chocolate, like honey, were prized and noted 4,000 years ago.

Eating chocolate, like honey, can help enhance the immune system, lower the risk of heart disease, cancer, diabetes—even obesity—and boost longevity. Chocolate, like honey, is chock-full of antioxidants. What's more, both supersweets can relieve dozens of ailments, including depression and high blood pressure, and rev up energy for both work and play.

Honey and chocolate have a lot in common, especially if it's quality dark chocolate and raw, natural honey. Both forbidden foods—because they contain sugar—play a role in the heart-healthy Mediterranean diet (savored in moderation) and lifestyle and are an integral part of life in Italy and other countries. And when they are teamed together you get a double delight, not to forget antioxidants.

Okay, enough about sweet things and why they're sweet. How about a chocolate honey candy recipe? I tried this recipe one day when I was craving dark chocolate. Instead of using peppermint I used a potpourri of creamed honeys: apricot, blackberry, peach, and raspberry. Also, I used 60 percent cocoa content chocolate chips.

Honey Chocolate Mint Patties

❖ ❖ ❖

1 cup (6 ounces) semi-sweet chocolate chips, divided
½ cup whipped honey

½ teaspoon peppermint extract
Powdered sugar for dusting (optional)

Line baking sheet with waxed or parchment paper; set aside. Place half of chocolate in small, microwave-safe container. Microwave on "High" (100 percent), 1 to 2 minutes, until melted; stir until smooth. Drop a heaping ½ teaspoon of chocolate on paper. With back of spoon, spread chocolate on paper to 2 inches. Repeat to form 24 circles; chill until firm. In small bowl, blend honey with peppermint extract. Spoon a scant teaspoon of honey mixture onto each circle. Freeze until firm. Microwave remaining chocolate; using same procedure. Spread a heaping ½ teaspoon of chocolate on top of each candy, making sure honey is completely covered with chocolate; chill until firm. Patties may be stored in refrigerator. Dust with powered sugar before serving, if desired. Makes 24 servings.

(*Source:* National Honey Board.)

Speaking of sweet combos, in part 5: "Tea and Honey," you'll learn that the world of teas with honeys is like a great place with an amazing must-do roller coaster in Honeyland. The wide range of teas and honeys is amazing. Teaming these two old-world superfoods with healing powers is one more secret to staying healthy, maintaining your weight, stalling age-related diseases, and living a longer, happier life.

Un-bee-lievable Healing Hints to Catch

✓ Honey-related products are becoming more and more popular and are better for your health.
✓ Beware of products that boast "includes honey" and note other ingredients, too, and see where honey places on the product label. The closer to first, the better.

- ✓ Honey drinks with vinegar are in demand both in the United States and around the globe, especially in Asian countries.
- ✓ The French paradox exists and makes sense . . . The French people who do indulge in chocolate, nuts, ice cream, and honey in small portions on a regular basis and who get a move on daily—plus drink antioxidant-rich red wine in moderation—stay healthy and live longer.
- ✓ Both honey and dark chocolate have been found to contain antioxidants—compounds linked to increasing heart health, lowering risk of developing cancers, and boosting longevity.
- ✓ Pairing the right chocolate with the right honey in desserts is an art that can be learned for your palate's and health's sake.

PART 5

TEA AND HONEY

Tea(s) with Your Honey

When the girl returned, some hours later, she carried a tray with a cup of fragrant tea steaming on it; and a plate piled with very hot buttered toast, cut thick, very brown on both sides, with the butter running through the holes in it in great golden drops, like honey from the honeycomb.

—Kenneth Grahame,
The Wind in the Willows[1]

After my freewheeling days in sunny Southern California, from the multiple beaches to mountains and the desert—places honey bees are found—I took a trip to Catalina Island, west of Long Beach. The destination was the rustic Zane Grey Pueblo Hotel overlooking Avalon Bay and the quaint town touted for its cosmopolitan feel. Inside the desert gold room—the study of the American novelist—was a sweet treat.

The first morning, I walked down the stairs to the charming swimming pool area overlooking Avalon Bay. I was greeted with a continental breakfast, including fresh apples, bananas, oranges, coffee, and tea. My dream in paradise was disturbed like a bee colony being bothered by an intruder when I couldn't find it: "Where's the honey?" I said out loud to myself. Eating toast and sipping tea without nature's sweetest gift is similar to being served a slice of hot apple pie without vanilla ice cream. But I survived.

These days, at Lake Tahoe, I do get my Mediterranean fix without leaving the sierra. It's the Mediterranean foods, the resort where I swim, and honey, the common sweetener of the Mediterranean diet, that keep me at peace without traveling like a forager. And a cup of tea and honey maintains that Mediterranean feeling. . . .

HONEY (AND TEA), LET'S FALL IN LOVE

For centuries, people all around the world have enjoyed the simple, soothing pleasures of a good cup of tea with a good teaspoon of honey, and nowadays there is more reason to do so. Black and green teas are not only good tasting, especially with honey, but together they pack a punch of nutritional and health benefits.

Herbal teas come from a variety of plants other than the tea plant. They are made from leaves, berries, flowers, fruits, and the bark of herbs and spices. Although most herbal teas do not contain the antioxidant properties of "real" tea—black, green, oolong, white, and red—paired with antioxidant-rich honey they do possess a wallop of good-for-you compounds that can enhance your health and well-being.

Another new feature on the Mediterranean diet pyramid is the addition of herbs, like spices, for reasons of both health and taste. Also, herbs contribute to the Mediterranean dishes.

Medical doctors, nutritionists, scientists, and bee-keepers are now confirming what healers have been saying since biblical times—teas and honeys have a variety of healing powers.

SWEET SIPS

Here are my six favorite tea and honey marriages—but there are infinite combinations for both you and me to try. There is no right or wrong combination and what's sweet to you makes honey-tea beverages a sweet sip.

1 **Black Tea:** The first tea I was introduced to was basic black tea—which does contain caffeine—and I have enjoyed it plain but realized it did need a sweet flavor boost to it. Also, Earl Grey and English breakfast teas (perfect for an Irish breakfast, complete with fried potatoes, scrambled eggs, and scones) are part of the black tea group.

   Best Honey Matches: Basswood has a distinct flavor that I've used in plain yogurt for a rich flavor and it can give black tea a kick, too. Sourwood boasts a caramel taste that can make a common black tea come to life with taste. Earl Grey teams well with avocado, blueberry, and eucalyptus honeys, too. It's more exotic and exciting than just using a simple all-purpose clover honey that comes without pleasant surprises.

2 **Green Tea:** Touted for its wide array of health virtues, this Asian tea does contain caffeine, like

black tea, but not as much. It's an acquired taste and that's where honey comes into play, so you can get the best of taste and nutritional benefits.

Best Honey Matches: Blueberry honey has a fruity taste that can give a nice kick to green tea, not the most flavorful tea. Sage honey is mild, a California favorite of mine that brings out the best of green tea.

3 **Fruit Tea:** Welcome to lemon, orange, rose hip, and apple teas. These fruity teas are sweet and sometimes tart, which calls for a honey sidekick.

Best Honey Matches: Mild-flavored honeys such as sage and alfalfa bring out the best in fruit teas because they don't overpower the fruity taste but maintain the integrity of the fruit flavor.

4 **Herbal Tea:** Herbal teas come from a variety of plants other than the tea plant. They are made from leaves, berries, flowers, fruits, and the bark of herbs and spices.

Although most herbal teas do not contain the antioxidant properties of "real" tea, they do possess other good-for-you compounds that can enhance your health and well-being. There is a wide range of herbal teas, including ginseng, cinnamon, licorice, and mint.

Rooibos (roy-boss) is the "new" herbal tea on the block—often called red tea. Like green and black teas, this tea contains antioxidants that make it heart-healthy and immunity enhancing—and it's caffeine free.

Best Honey Matches: Earthy and warm herbal teas go well with mild alfalfa, clover, orange blossom, and sage honeys—common honeys that complement distinct herbal flavors.

5 **Oolong Tea:** This tea, popular in Asian countries, contains the health perks of both black and green teas. A robust-flavored tea that can have a sweet taste lends itself to different honeys.

Best Honey Matches: Oolong, not a tea familiar to me, was easy to try with a friendly California orange blossom honey with its citrusy sweet taste. Another oolong mate is tupelo honey with its light amber color and herbal, fruity flavors.

6 **White Tea:** And last but not least, welcome to this pale tea. Found in China, it is believed to rank number one for its antioxidants. It's a bit sweet and mellow. It's the new tea on the block for tea lovers.

Best Honey Matches: Fireweed honey is light colored and smooth, like white tea—the two complement each other. Wildflower, one of my favorite mild honeys, also goes nicely with white tea.

As a devout tea drinker, I believe your choice of honey and tea is a personal one—like pairing dark chocolate with different fruits, herbs, and spices. The selection also depends on the season to your mood. But popular and friendly honeys, such as clover and orange blossom, are suitable anytime, anyplace, because they are not too strong and will not overpower teas—all types—and you can't go wrong for yourself or if you're serving other people.

Travels with Honey (and Teas)

Tea and honey have played a starring role in my life, decade after decade. . . .

In my twenties: I recall in Hollywood, California, I was a carefree unpublished author. My best friend and I would frequent a popular hotel/coffee shop on Sunset Boulevard and order spicy cinnamon tea and pair it with honey while we waited for our tossed green salads and to be discovered.

In my thirties: In San Francisco, as a penniless graduate student, after class and on-spec writing assignments I'd visit my dentist in the Financial District. Tea was offered in the waiting room. I'd sip orange pekoe with a bit of honey to calm dental jitters until I was called into the dental chair.

In my forties: During this passage of my life, I was a busy magazine journalist. Black tea with its caffeine content was the drink of choice as I met deadline after deadline. Also, in between writing, looking for Mr. Soul Mate was on my plate during tea-and-honey blind dates. The tea kept me centered and coming home to my best friend: my loyal Labrador.

In my fifties: I live as a solo author-intuitive in the sierra, chamomile tea and honey my trusty companions. In the summer it's citrus tea with sage honey; in the fall it's herbal tea and alfalfa tea; in the winter it's black and green tea with orange blossom honey; in the spring it's fruit teas and clover honey.

As I look back on the years of tea and honey, it's clear that this beverage has brought me comfort. Several years ago, before I penned the book *The Man Who Predicts Earthquakes: Jim Berkland, Maverick Geologist* (Boulder, CO: Sentient Publications, 2006), the nature-loving scientist paid me a visit at my cabin at Lake Tahoe. For five hours we chatted about his past and present earthquake predictions. In between bites of cheese, French bread, and cheesecake and sips of chamomile tea, we discussed what was shaking around the nation. Like old friends, Jim and I discussed fault lines we had experienced. Today, if I served these foods I'd give them a worldly twist with honey varietals in my pantry. I'd provide avocado honey for the cheese and French bread. The cheesecake would be drizzled with a blueberry or lemon honey, and for the calming chamomile? I'd offer a cinnamon and clove tea or orange blossom from California. The potpourri of honeys would have added an earthy sophistication to the European-style buffet I created for the man who predicts quakes and taught me how to tune in to my intuition and do it, too. Thank goodness for tea and honey—the two friends that have kept me company, and calm and skinny, throughout the years.

HOW TEETOTALERS STAY SLIM

Spa nutritionists will tell you that drinking a soothing hot beverage is similar to having a hot cup of soup before a meal. It satisfies your appetite and you'll eat less. A hot liquid can fill you up, not out.

Herbal teas with honey are caffeine free, unlike black and green tea, coffee, and soda. If you max out on caffeinated beverages it can cause your blood sugar to spike and plummet like an amusement park ride, leaving you feeling tired and cranky or likely to reach for more caffeine or junk food to get another quick pick-me-up. This does not happen with soothing teas.

Some of the best skinny teas work to help women and men get and stay slim because they contain herbs, including marshmallow root, dandelion, and parsley, that can help stimulate water loss and/or beat bloat. Then, if you turn to the weight loss tea superstar—green tea, a known fat fighter—you'll be on the path to real weight loss.

Not only can drinking teas help you to lose water weight, but the soothing beverage can also calm and uplift your spirits. This connection between destressing and teas is another slim-down perk that is used at health spas around the world and by the rich and famous. Tea breaks give you a minivacation to replenish your body, mind, and spirit. Here, take a look at this recipe, straight from a chef who knows spa food and spa teas.

Rosehip and Cranberry Tea

❖ ❖ ❖

2 cups water
1½ cups cranberry
    juice
1 clove
2 rose hip tea bags,
    or 2 rose hip-
    blend tea bags

2 tablespoons clover
    honey
2 orange slices for
    garnish

Combine the water, cranberry juice, and clove in a medium-size pot set over medium heat. Bring to a simmer.

Using a spoon, remove the clove from the cranberry juice. Place the rose hip tea bags into a warmed teapot, pour in the hot cranberry-water mixture, stir in the honey, and steep for 5 to 7 minutes. Pour into mugs, garnish with orange slices and serve.

(*Source:* Reprinted with permission from *The Golden Door Cooks Light & Easy*, by Chef Michel Stroot, published by Gibbs Smith © 2003.)

Speaking of tea and good health, in part 6: "Honey Cures" you'll get a taste of how honey and teaming different types are the natural path to tending to annoying and chronic health ailments, including allergies, colds, sore throats, and so much more.

Un-bee-lievable Healing Hints to Catch

- ✓ Medical doctors and scientists are now confirming what herbalists have known for years—tea and honey have a variety of healing powers.
- ✓ Throughout history, ancient cultures have used herbs and honeys to stay healthy and live longer.
- ✓ Antioxidant-rich "real" teas, including black, green, oolong, and red, paired with darker honeys provide extra healing properties.
- ✓ Tea and honey pairing is a personal preference, but there are matches that are popular, including black tea: basswood, clover; green tea: sage; fruit tea: sage, alfalfa; herbal tea: clover, orange blossom; oolong tea: orange blossom, tupelo; white tea: wildflower.

PART 6

HONEY CURES

Home Remedies from Your Kitchen

*The fruit of bees is desired by all, and is equally
sweet to kings and beggars and it is not only
pleasing but profitable and healthful; it sweetens
mouths, cures their wounds, and conveys remedies
to inward ulcers.*

—Saint Ambrose[1]

Like a wayward honey bee spreading its wings and re-
turning to its colony, I headed back home with my dog,
Stone Fox, to Northern California. But we got side-
tracked. On the way we ended up in Fresno, Central
California—a honey bee haven. I was a nanny. My job
was to tend to two kids and one giant, cumbersome
Saint Bernard. It was a semi-rural neighborhood in the
hot summertime. On my days off I'd flee on a 10-speed
bicycle. My dog and I moved wild and free through the
orange groves—a place where honey bees worked. I

picked up oranges under the fruit trees and took them home to use the fruits of my labor.

In the kitchen, as usual, I found myself like a worker in its hive. Clad in blue-jean overalls, barefoot, and golden brown from the sun, I'd play road songs, such as "Ventura Highway" and "Born to Be Wild," and do a honey bee waggle dance—but I was all alone. I created fresh orange juice Popsicles sweetened with a bit of local fresh orange blossom honey—used in my home remedies. The honey helped soothe dry skin, insect bites, PMS, and sunburn—all ailments I endured while enduring Central California, a place I didn't feel was home.

Discovering home cures, like these, can give you peace of mind—and often work to cure common ailments, which will make you a believer that your kitchen cabinet is like a medicine cabinet.

Cures from Your Kitchen

I'll describe 50 common health ailments alphabetically and provide amazing at-home honey cures. I include tried-and-true folk remedies, real-life stories, scientific studies, and medical experts' words of honey wisdom—and my own experiences with honey. But caution, consult your health-care practitioner before putting to work any honey cure.

1 **ACNE (Brush off blemishes):** Red dots on your face, back, and shoulders are the scourge of the young and beautiful. But adults aren't immune from adult acne or flare-ups. As a teen, I blamed my mom and dad for my blotchy face. (Genes and hormones can play a role in acne.) I turned to gooey Clearasil cream and smelly Stridex pads

and went to war like a fearless Indian using war paint and getting ready to go to battle. But my efforts didn't work.

I ended up going to a dermatologist and using a potent topical medicine. After applying more rather than less (I don't follow instructions) I ended up tying a navy blue bandana across my forehead to hide the unsightly blotch—and was grateful for the hippie fashion trend. If I had known that there was a gentler cure to clear up my face, I would have used it in a heartbeat.

What Honey Rx to Use: Put a dab of honey (a darker variety such as manuka) on blemishes. Repeat twice per day. Sip a cup of chamomile tea to chill—and drink 6- to 8-ounce glasses of water daily and stay clear of the empty nutrition of sugary beverages with caffeine.

Why You'll Bee Happy: It's the antibacterial compounds in honey that work to help fight redness, inflammation, and infection and dry up the blemish. Manuka honey is antioxidant rich, which can help give you a clearer, smoother complexion. "As a teenager," recalls one honey lover, "I would smear raw, organic honey on my face and did it after I came home from school, every day." Two months later, he recalls seeing sweet results—a 50 percent clearer complexion. The credit goes to using the right "type" of honey—not processed kinds.

2 **ALLERGIES (Stop seasonal misery):** Dealing with annoying acne is no picnic, but sneezing, a runny nose, and coughing can ruin an indoor or outdoor event, thanks to seasonal pollen. Every year when the yellow pollen arrives like an uninvited

visitor at Lake Tahoe I hold a tissue in one hand and am on the phone to a pharmacist with the other. I am always on a mission to find the natural remedy to stop my sniffles.

What Honey Rx to Use: Try eating a tablespoon of locally produced honey. Proponents of honey tell me that your immune system will get used to the local pollen in it (it should be within a 50-mile radius from where you live).

Why You'll Bee Happy: By taking the honey cure, you may lose your allergy symptoms. Or not. It's worth the effort and is less pricey than a visit to the doctor or an allergist. Also, honey is a natural remedy and doesn't come with unknown side effects linked to allergy medications or pricey shots. One summer day, I looked outside and the Tahoe yellow pollen was everywhere—on cars, trees, and the ground. I started putting honey (not just the local alfalfa variety) in my tea, yogurt, and baking. Two days later, my sniffles were history. Whether it was coincidence or a honey cure doesn't matter. It worked.

If you have mild respiratory problems, from allergies to asthma, honey may enhance the immune system to build up a better arsenal against airborne allergens—and help you breathe easier. Honey enthusiasts like D. C. Jarvis, M.D., believe honeycomb is excellent for treating certain breathing problems. The honey prescription, according to him, was chewing honeycomb, which may line the entire breathing tract.[2]

Also, eating honey on a daily basis was recommended: "As far as I have been able to learn, Vermont folk medicine uses honeycomb as a desensitizing agent; from the results obtained by its use it appears to be anti-allergic in its action." Dr. Jarvis gives credit to the honey bees.[3]

Beekeepers tell me that honey may help allergies linked to trees and ragweed—the culprit in hay fever and its irritating symptoms during spring and autumn months and often right before. If mold and food allergens are bothering you, honey is not going to be your allergy cure. As beekeepers are busy at work selling local honey to allergy sufferers, I am busy including all types of honeys in my diet because I want to be covered in both seasons. And if honey can help me cope with congestion and sneezing, I'm in. While further research is needed, I'm not going to wait for scientists to go to their lab rats for a go-ahead. More honey, please.

3 ANEMIA (Iron up): Allergies can affect people of all ages, but anemia may be more of a problem for people who are dieting or vegetarians who are not getting sufficient iron. Simply put, anemia is a lack of red blood cells and hemoglobin, the protein in red blood cells that moves oxygen to cells in your body. The symptoms can include feeling tired and light-headed.

What Honey Rx to Use: Try incorporating a dark honey, such as buckwheat, in your daily diet. Pair it with Mediterranean iron-rich foods, including fish, seafood, apricots, and figs.

Why You'll Bee Happy: If you're borderline iron deficient, you need to pump more iron into your body. The daily recommended value of iron is 18 milligrams. If you are borderline anemic, you can boost your iron intake by increasing iron-rich foods and dark honeys containing iron, which can help boost red blood cells in the body.

4　**ANXIETY (Beat the jitters monster):** Anemia sometimes comes with warnings of symptoms, but when anxiety hits (often worsened by stress) you know it like when an earthquake strikes. Anxiety can wreak havoc on your nervous system and up your odds of experiencing heart disease, stress eating, and other chronic health problems.

What Honey Rx to Use: If you're under pressure and feeling high anxiety or sense a stressful event is in the works, make a cup of chamomile tea. Put in 1 teaspoon of your favorite honey. Repeat twice a day as needed.

Why You'll Bee Happy: Honey—all varietals—is touted by folk medicine healers for its calming effects. The natural superfood can help soothe your nerves rather than put you in higher anxiety mode. The relief it provides may be due to its multiple vitamin B content—antistress vitamins. Pairing it with calming tea or milk (which is rich in tryptophan, an essential amino acid that helps to alleviate feelings of anxiety and stress) can help you to chill. So next time you want to relax, one of the best cures is carbohydrates—and the fastest worker to giving you a chill pill is nature's sweet honey.

5　**BAD BREATH (Freshen up your mouth):** Feeling anxious if your breath is not as sweet as it should be? Bad breath can be linked to a variety of causes, from a bad tooth, gingivitis, and eating onions to sinusitis.

What Honey Rx to Use: Try 1 teaspoon of honey in a cup of herbal tea. Repeat as needed.

Why You'll Bee Happy: If you are suffering from postnasal drip, drinking hot tea with honey (which has antibacterial properties) can help clear up mucus and that'll help sweeten your mouth. Drinking a cup of honey and chamomile tea will also soothe inflamed gum tissue because of its anti-inflammatory properties. Onions, like any pungent food, will take a while to fade out, but a honey and tea remedy may offer a quick fix. And if you have a tooth that needs attention, seek it and save that sweet tooth.

6 **BEDSORES (Stave off a sore spot):** Halitosis can be a sensitive issue for folks, but bedsores are another pain (at any age). If you've been a caretaker for an elderly person (or if you're the one who is dealing with bedsores due to being bedridden) you're aware of the potential of getting and coping with pain and potential infection.

What Honey Rx to Use: Try applying a medicinal honey, such as manuka, on the sore. Repeat in the morning and night. Follow directions on the product you use, because there are different forms available.

Why You'll Bee Happy: Scientific research proves honey contains powerful antibacterial compounds, which can help soothe inflammation and heal sores—all kinds. So, if this tried-and-true all-natural cure works, it will provide a sigh of relief and honey power will be a welcomed change for the better.

7 BED-WETTING (Catch a break): Coping with bedsores can be a challenge, but so is not knowing what to do when your child wets the bed. This is not a new or abnormal problem, but it does take patience to find the right cure. I recall in the film *2012* the mother pointed out to her husband that yes, their seven-year-old daughter still wet the bed and gave him the bed gear to deal—as we see her at the store buying more nighttime diapers. But wetting the bed doesn't have to be the end of the world, because in the real world there is the honey cure that may really work wonders for you and your child.

What Honey Rx to Use: The Vermont country doctor D. C. Jarvis recommends 1 teaspoon of honey at mealtime and before bed. Avoid giving water a few hours before bedtime.[4]

Why You'll Bee Happy: One reason why this cure may do the trick is because honey contains tryptophan, an amino acid that can relax the nervous system and allow sleep to be without interruptions. A dry bed will make you and a child feel empowered, boost confidence, and give incentive to continue the old-fashioned remedy until the mission is accomplished without super sci-fi gimmicks.

8 BLAHS (Try a sweet pick-me-up): Bed-wetting to blahs, both woes can take a toll on one's well-being—body and mind. If the bills are stacking up and you're working hard for the money or are out of work, you may be feeling down-and-out like an ailing honey bee. Or maybe family members or friends are unhappy? Is the cat or dog sick? Temporary setbacks and stressors in life can zap our

Pollyanna type of mood. Can there be a kitchen cure that can make you feel not all gloom and doom?

What Honey Rx to Use: Put lemon juice from one lemon into an 8-ounce cup of water with ice or cup of hot water. Add 1 teaspoon of wildflower honey (it has medicinal properties) and stir, sip, and wait for a change in your spirit. Repeat as necessary.

Why You'll Bee Happy: Make way, sugary sodas and caffeinated java! This honey cure has fructose and glucose that are absorbed in the bloodstream faster than you can say, "I feel under the weather." It's a natural jolt to your nervous system and naturally refreshing, so it provides a worker bee pick-me-up. Think a buzzing honey bee on a wildflower in the springtime.

9 **BONE LOSS (Prevent brittle bone disease):** Osteoporosis, with the loss of bone density, is often thought of as an older person's disease, but just like feeling blah, it can strike at any age. Bone loss can happen for many reasons, including if you have a small, thin frame (like I do), a family history of osteoporosis, are postmenopausal (like I am), are sedentary (as an author I am, but I exercise daily), and eat a diet low in dairy products and other sources of calcium (I am a yogurt and low-fat milk addict).

What Honey Rx to Use: Include a teaspoon of honey (in pure liquid form or bee pollen) in a cup of plain yogurt or smoothie with low-fat milk each day.

Why You'll Bee Happy: Honey contains calcium and B vitamins—including vitamin B_6. The bone-building nutrient plays a big role in bone metabolism because it's necessary for hydrochloric acid production, which is required in calcium absorption. Best food sources include poultry and fish. These foods can be teamed with honeys, such as glazes. (See chapter 18: "Ciao, Honey!") to enjoy the variety of recipes that can help you maintain strong bones.

Boron deficiency may also be connected with an increased risk for bone loss. Boron, like vitamin B_6, helps metabolism of calcium and magnesium. Boron is richest in honey and fruits, especially apples, pears, grapes, dates, raisins, and peaches, and in legumes, soybeans, and nuts—all of which the honey bee pollinates.

Also, use whole foods rather than processed ones. This way you'll not lose nature's nutrients. Whole foods include whole grains (brown rice and whole-grain flour), which you should use instead of white flour products. Use fresh vegetables, rather than canned. Opt for beans, fresh fruits, nuts, and seeds. All of these nutrient-dense good foods (strong bones need more than B vitamins and boron) can be enhanced with good honey to maintain strong bones.

A Back-to-Nature Bee Girl

Meet Angela Ysseldyk (www.beepollen-buzz.com), nicknamed Bee Girl. She grew up on the Dutchman's Gold bee farm in Carlisle, Ontario, Canada: "When I was a young girl growing up on a bee farm, my mom made sure I was fed plenty of raw honey and bee pollen. I can even remember sprinkling bee pollen granules on my home-made granola!"

Sweet honey was the folk medicine of choice in the house when she or one of her four siblings got a cold. "It was raw bee propolis for us and not antibiotics," says the pro-bee girl who is buzzing about the fact that her mother raised her holistically. The diet of the farm for her family was whole, unprocessed foods, and there was no junk food allowed in the house.

As time passed, Angela got her calling to teach people about good nutrition, supplements, and organic food. So, the next stop was attending the Institute of Holistic Nutrition in Toronto. The end result: One bee girl blossomed into a Registered Holistic Nutritionist who teaches people at a health-food store about the healing powers of honey and its healing by-products, including royal jelly—the gifts of bees and fed to larvae and virgin queens and queen bees.

10 **BURNS (Baby skin burns):** Bone loss doesn't hurt until you fall, but a burn can be painful immediately. When I was a kid I recall my mom was frying chicken, the oil splattered, and she burned her arm. It was butter that she used to soothe the inflammation and pain. It was a big deal because I saw the popping oil and small stovetop fire. These days, if I experienced a cooking burn I'd try a different quick home cure.

What Honey Rx to Use: Apply manuka honey or a first-aid lotion with manuka honey on the burned area.

Why You'll Bee Happy: The Vermont country doctor D. C. Jarvis recommends honey for burns because it can relieve the painful smarting, stave off blisters, and speed up the healing process of the burned area.[5]

11 **CAVITIES (Kiss off dental caries):** Like skin burns, holes in your teeth can stress you out and hurt, too. Since honey is a sweetener, it is believed that it can cause visits to the dentist and drill. But hold off on laughing gas, because these days medical researchers believe that the right type of honey can actually stave off cavities.

What Honey Rx to Use: Opt for the darker type of honey when choosing the home cure to include in your healthy-teeth diet regime.

Why You'll Bee Happy: Honey guru Joe Traynor says the fact is, "sucrose rots your teeth; honey is good for teeth." He explains that tooth decay requires sucrose to form plaque (the sticky stuff that forms on tooth enamel). We know granulated white sugar is 100 percent sucrose, but honey is made of glucose and fructose—and the antibacterial properties of honey help keep tooth decay at bay.

Research suggests Traynor could be right. The honey bee's by-product may be useful in treatment of cavities. The extract of propolis was looked at for its antimicrobial activities. The findings, published in the *African Journal of Biotechnology*, show that the "bee glue" has a strong antimicrobial action and hints that it may be useful in the treatment of dental cavities.[6]

The Queen Bee's Honey Tips for Cold and Flu Season

In my pantry are bee pollen, propolis, royal jelly, and other gifts of the honey bee—and from Dutchman's Gold natural honey and maple products. Dazed and confused, I contacted a few folks in the honey world, but nobody said that they had tried the royal jelly or other bee products. Then, I contacted my local health-food store. I was told that they do carry these special by-products and that they are used for medicinal use—not like honey varietals we put to work in drizzling on cheeses and yogurt and in cooking and baking.

Erika Van Alten of Dutchman's Gold has more than two dozen years of experience with the healing powers of honey, and she shed some light to me on what honey prescription to use when you're not sure which one to use. . . .

"The sound of a cough from a cold is a rare memory from my childhood; however, I do recall the sweet taste of honey and the morning rituals of eating bee pollen. . . .

My mother, Annie, the Queen Bee and Dr. Mom, was quick to

quell the onset of cold and flu viruses with the application of therapeutic bee products in our family hive. We used honey to ease many illnesses but also other products that the bees work hard to collect such as bee propolis, royal jelly, and bee pollen. These products have been applied to prevent and heal disease and maintain health for thousands of years.

Dry and sore throats: pure honeycomb; buckwheat honey; honey sticks. *Fever, flu, cold, or bronchial infection:* propolis throat spray; propolis tincture; raw propolis chunks; propolis capsules. *Stress cold:* fresh royal jelly; royal jelly capsules. *Immune booster and energizer:* bee pollen. Try a tablespoon in a smoothie or all on its own.

12 **COLD SORES (Good riddance to the ouch):** A common woe can pay you an untimely visit in the form of an unsightly cold sore—both come uninvited. Imagine this all-too-familiar scenario: You wake up in the morning before a big event. In the mirror a red, swollen cold sore or fever blister around the mouth gives you a rude awakening. It's good to know these sores are not life threatening. Yes, you'll survive the red blister(s) caused by the herpes simplex virus, and they will go away by themselves after several days. The

good news is, there may be a gentle way to speed up their departure and your healing process.

What Honey Rx to Use: Dab honey (manuka is recommended, but any honey may work) on top of the cold sore. Repeat two to three times each day.

Why You'll Bee Happy: There are different antibacterial compounds in honey that can help fight skin sores. Jane from New Britain, Connecticut, decided to give the cure-all healer a try on a cold sore that had just begun to redden on her upper lip. "I've used over-the-counter products which help . . . but not until the cold sore has bloomed in a big, ugly mess on my face." The honey (from The Manuka Bees Company) did its job in stopping this cold sore. Two days later, the cold sore was dormant, like a volcano warning that had fizzled.

13 CONSTIPATION (Get regular): Cold sores are painful and not pretty, but being irregular can make you feel ugly. Irregularity can be due to eating less, resting more. Also, not eating enough fiber-rich foods or drinking enough water, a change in climate and environment, as well as not staying physically active can wreak havoc on your digestive system. But honey comes to the rescue.

What Honey Rx to Use: Before bedtime or in the morning, try 1 teaspoon of honey in a glass of warm water with fresh lemon. Or, if you prefer, try that honey cure in a fresh cup of strong java, and your irregular woe will soon be history.

Why You'll Bee Happy: Because honey contains a healthy dose of sugar, which can cause a mild laxative effect, it may help induce regularity in some people, especially sensitive individuals. (Yes, honey has been my sweet friend during irregular spells.)

14 **COUGH (Outfox irritating hacking):** Irregularity and coughs can interrupt our life as we like it. No matter what age you are, a cough is another unwelcome visitor and can make you feel terrible. Let's face it, cough medicine can be pricey, doesn't taste good, and may or may not do its job. Also, what if it's in the middle of the night or the drugstore is closed?

What Honey Rx to Use: A teaspoon of buckwheat honey is recommended before bed. Or you can make syrup of 1 teaspoon lemon juice, 1 teaspoon honey, and 1 teaspoon apple cider vinegar. Repeat each remedy as needed.

Why You'll Bee Happy: Twentieth-century scientists have proven that honey can stop a cough just like cough medicine does—and even better. A group of Penn State College of Medicine researchers discovered that honey may offer parents an effective and safe alternative. The findings showed that buckwheat at bedtime was more powerful for curing a cough in children than dextromethorphan (not recommended for children less than six years old), a cough suppressant found in over-the-counter cold medications. But note, honey is not to be given to children under the age of one due to the ill effects of botulism.[7]

What's more, Dr. D. C. Jarvis notes that honey will act as a sedative to the nervous system. It also will attract and hold fluid when you're sleeping.[8]

15 DEPRESSION (Defeat the blues): Now that the kids or you aren't coughing, the bad news, according to the National Institute of Mental Health, is that about 10 percent of Americans wade through at least one bout of melancholy misery sometime during their lives. The victim list of depression sufferers includes Virginia Woolf and Ludwig van Beethoven, as well as everyday people including truck drivers, clerks, salespeople, actors, and musicians. No one is immune.

What Honey Rx to Use: Try a spoonful of honey. Or opt for bee pollen, which is rich in B_1, B_2, B_6, and B_{12}—and contains 18 amino acids. Take it on a daily basis beginning with a few granules, working up to a teaspoon as needed. If you're feeling down, don't give up on the honey cure. Although depression can prove to be a depressingly complicated ailment, daily health habits can offset its effects. That means getting regular exercise (honey can help boost your stamina), eating healthy (refer to chapter 6: "The Mediterranean Sweetener"), and getting adequate sleep to help treat mild depression may defeat those blues.

Why You'll Bee Happy: There is light at the end of the dark tunnel for gloom-and-doom feelings. Research shows that diet and lifestyle can lower your risk of depression—and honey plays a role in feeling upbeat. Depression has been linked to lack of the B vitamins. These vitamins are often involved in the production of energy, and a large component of depression may encompass the inability to get out of bed and deal with the ups and downs of the world.

Amino acids, also found in honey and bee pollen, are the vital building blocks of protein and may also help improve mood. The amino acids are used by the body to construct brain chemicals that help alleviate depression. So are we feeling a bit happier?

16 **DETOXIFICATION (Say good-bye to toxins):** Feeling down is a drag, and when your body is polluted that'll drag you down, too. No matter what season you're in, it's healthful to give your body a minivacation from too many unhealthy toxins. I'm talking about junk food (i.e., empty-calorie processed foods), caffeine, and high-fat foods. A minidetox minifast is healthier than a total fast because it's not a major shock to your system. You can still eat water-dense fruits and vegetables to help you to cleanse your system, along with dark honey, which can sweeten the goal of detoxing your body, mind, and spirit.

What Honey Rx to Use: Mix a teaspoon or two of stronger-flavored, antioxidant-rich honeys (such as buckwheat or leatherwood) paired with 1 teaspoon of unfiltered apple cider vinegar in cold or hot water each morning before breakfast.

Why You'll Bee Happy: By pairing honey with a minifast of fresh fruits, vegetables, and 6- to 8-ounce glasses of water, you will help to give your organs a rest from toxins in foods and cleanse and rejuvenate your body. Also, the honey will give you an energetic buzz to help you stay physical as well as stave off cravings for sweets.

17 **DIARRHEA (Leave behind a pesky problem):** A bout of the runs can be triggered by many things,

including a detoxifying minifast, antibiotics, or eating a food gone bad. Everyone at one time or another has experienced this miserable visitor and wants it to go away ASAP.

What Honey Rx to Use: Try 1 cup of calming chamomile or ginger tea with 1 teaspoon of honey three times per day.

Why You'll Bee Happy: Personally, I stay clear of the anti-go tablets, because while they can work often irregularity may follow. Honey and tea, a soothing, natural remedy, is comforting and can help stop the urge to go and go. It works because honey is a quick and easy route to easing intestinal problems, as it coats the stomach lining. Team honey with yogurt, another probiotic that helps keep the "good" bacteria in your system. Both honey and yogurt boast antibacterial properties and probiotic effects—and get rid of the "bad" bacteria. It's a win-win end result.

18 DIGESTIVE PROBLEMS (Tame tummy drama):

Running to the bathroom or feeling the pain of colitis (inflammation of the colon) or irritable bowel syndrome (IBS: a spastic colon that has a mind of its own) can be a pain in the rear (pun intended). So, when your internal pipes are out of whack, that's a cue to turn to the friendly bacteria found in sweet honey (and in the future before as a sweet preventative measure).

What Honey Rx to Use: Take 1 tablespoon of manuka honey (less than 10 UMF), bee pollen, or propolis on an empty stomach. Or, if preferred, put 1 teaspoon honey in a cup of soothing ginger or peppermint tea.

Why You'll Bee Happy: Scientists in New Zealand found a cause of upset stomach is the bacteria strain *Helicobacter pylori.* A 5 percent solution of honey slowed the growth of the bacteria. Ingredients used were manuka honey (UMF 20+), bee pollen, and propolis.[9]

A study is good, but if it works for you it's great. Back in my college days, for instance, IBS paid me frequent visits. I saw a gastroenterologist. He took out a prescription pad and scribbled: "Drink water, eat fiber-rich foods, destress, and exercise." In retrospect, I realize he was spot-on. But in hindsight I sense he should have included honey on the at-home to-do list.

19 **ENERGY DRAIN (Beat low energy):** Getting your digestive system back on track is a good feeling, but then what if your energy plummets? Savannah Bee Company founder Ted turns to liquid gold—the good stuff. "I take a healthy-sized spoonful of bee pollen every day. It gives me a boost of energy and is packed with all of the vitamins and minerals you need," he says. "It is said that man can survive on bee pollen, water, and sunshine. It helps me stay healthy and hopeful."

What Honey Rx to Use: Each morning include a teaspoon of bee pollen in your breakfast. Go ahead and take it solo. Or try The Honey Association's Energy Drink recipe: ¼ pint orange juice, ¼ pint natural yogurt, 2 tablespoons clear honey. Place all the ingredients in a liquidizer and blend until smooth. Pour into two tall glasses. Serves two people.

Why You'll Bee Happy: Honey is a source of natural unrefined sugars and carbohydrates, which are easily absorbed by the body. That means, you'll get a quick energy boost with long-lasting effects. Athletes include it in their daily diets. It was even used by runners at the Olympic Games in ancient Greece. If a spoonful of honey every day can give you extra energy to do all of the things you want to do, whether it be work or play, it makes sense to give it a try. And eating honey beats drinking sodas with caffeine or coffee, which give you a lift but leave you with a rollercoaster ride of ups and downs until you get your next fix. Stick with the honey bee's energy prescription.

20 **EYE HEALTH (Guard your eyes):** Feeling energized is a good thing, but having good eyesight is not to be taken for granted, either. I've had two middle-aged friends who fell victim to macular degeneration (deterioration of the macula in the eye, which can lead to blindness). Eyesight is a precious thing and often we forget how important it is until our own eyes are affected in one way or another.

What Honey Rx to Use: Include dark honeys in your daily diet teamed with antioxidant-rich fruits and vegetables.

Why You'll Bee Happy: Holistic doctors believe that flavonoids in foods can protect your eye health. We know that darker honeys contain antioxidants and when included in the daily diet couldn't hurt your eyes—but, of course, large government-funded scientific studies have not been done to prove consuming honey can help eye disorders. But *Honey: The Gourmet Medicine* author Joe Traynor points out how a small group of people with conjunctivitis applied honey under the lower eyelid as any eye ointment would be applied. Improvement was the end result, with Traynor saying that it may be the flavonoids in honey that have the properties to access the lens. He adds, "Antioxidant and osmotic properties of honey could also be a factor. Certainly the potential benefits of honey to treat cataracts deserve more study."

21 **FIBROMYALGIA (Lose the aches and pains):** Maintaining healthy eyes is a big deal, and so is keeping aches and pains at bay. If you've got chronic pain in the muscles and soft tissues surrounding joints, fatigue, and tenderness at specific sites in the body, you may have fibromyalgia syndrome or fibrositis. Today, medical people get it: They acknowledge the pain linked to the nervous system and there is relief provided from both conventional medicine and nature.

What Honey Rx to Use: Try 1 teaspoon of honey in a cup of hot tea three times per day. For relieving tight muscles, try a massage with a honey and milk moisturizing cream and/or a hot tub soak.

Why You'll Bee Happy: Honey is an energizing liquid that can give you a lift so you'll be more apt to be happy to exercise (which releases feel-good hormonal endorphins that'll lessen pain). Honey also contains anti-inflammatory properties, and both honey and tea, especially calming chamomile, can help you to fight stress and relax— a must-do. And the massage and hydrotherapy can help relax you and your muscles, which can reduce pain.

22 GALLSTONES (Prevent these little guys): Aches and pains in the muscles can come and go, just like gallstones. The adage "An ounce of prevention is worth a pound of cure" applies to this health ailment, which is more common in older people. Obesity, high cholesterol, and diabetes are all causes of gallstones, which can be a pain—but the good news is that you can be proactive and keep gallstones away with a healthful diet and lifestyle.

What Honey Rx to Use: Incorporate honey in your diet in a variety of ways and forms, including taking a teaspoon of the golden liquid each day, putting it in a cup of tea or low-fat milk, and drizzling it on nutrient-rich fruits and vegetables.

Why You'll Bee Happy: If you keep your weight in check, you up the odds of beating high cholesterol and diabetes. Honey used in moderation can help you stay clear of sweet junk food because it beats sweet cravings. It also gives you energy to stay physical, so you'll be more apt to rev up your metabolism and keep gallstones where they belong—out of your life.

23 HANGOVER (Sip away the blahs): Enjoying a healthful diet and lifestyle can help you avoid the dreaded hangover due to overindulgence of the spirits. A killer headache and the hypersensitivity to noise can be enough to cause you to seek a hangover helper that works, even if you have to find the nearest beehive and plead with the bees to let you have a bit of their brew.

What Honey Rx to Use: Try a spoonful or two of honey in a cup of hot chamomile or ginger tea. If you can stomach it, a piece of whole-grain toast spread with honey may be helpful, too.

Why You'll Bee Happy: Simply put, honey is chock-full of fructose and enzymes—a godsend to folks who overindulge in spirits of any kind one night or weekend because it can rev up the metabolism of alcohol, according to the *Honey: The Gourmet Medicine* author Joe Traynor.

24 HEADACHE (Bye-bye, pain): Hangovers and headaches—both are not to be taken with a grain of salt, because it can hurt oh, so bad. There are different types of headaches, tension, cluster, migraine, and sinus related. Personally, I am prone to sinus headaches, and these can be worse than getting a root canal.

What Honey Rx to Use: One cup of tea with 1 teaspoon of honey (the darker the varietal the better) is the remedy. Repeat as needed. Also, drink plenty of water and relax.

Why You'll Bee Happy: I went straight to the New York Headache Center in New York to ask Alexander Mauskop, M.D., if honey can help reduce tension headaches. "The way honey might work for tension headaches," he says, "is by treating hypoglycemia, which can cause tension and migraines, although it is more advisable to avoid getting hungry and eat small frequent meals." But caution is advised, because the good doctor warned that honey can cause reactive hypoglycemia and worsen the headache.

But can a teaspoon of dark antioxidant-rich honey or a cup of herbal tea with a teaspoon or two of honey help alleviate the ache? The doctor's response gave me hope for those pesky headaches that sneak up on me like a time traveler: "Yes, some antioxidants can help prevent headaches, as can magnesium and vitamin B." So, I quickly turned to a brewed cup of honey and tea (2 cups) and 2 teaspoons of light buckwheat honey, and yes, my sinus headache for the day did subside.

25 HEARTBURN (Get rid of the burn STAT): A pounding headache is a pain, but heartburn is like a monster relative that invades your body. Common culprits include tomato sauce, salsa, and alcoholic beverages. Time heals occasional heartburn, but why wait for the pain to go when you can use an all-natural cure that can provide relief perhaps sooner rather than later?

What Honey Rx to Use: Take 1 teaspoon of honey straight or try it with 1 cup of hot peppermint tea.

Why You'll Bee Happy: Move over, ROLAIDS! Honey has properties that naturally ease heartburn symptoms. Thanks to its effect on the bacteria associated with gastric ulcers, it's the "remedy for heartburn, gastric acid reflux or indigestion," says *The Honey Revolution* author Ron Fessenden, M.D. What's more, "honey consumed is rapidly diluted with saliva and gastric juices, so it destroys bacteria." Honey is also a probiotic, promoting the growth of the healthy bacteria in the gut.

26 HERPES (Soothe the sting): Heartburn comes and goes, as does herpes, a virus that plagues millions. It is a painful condition during outbreaks, but there are treatments that can speed up the process of flare-up, whether the sores are on the mouth or in the genital region.

What Honey Rx to Use: Apply a dab of medicinal honey to the affected area. Repeat every day until the sore or sores have healed.

Why You'll Bee Happy: Mainstream doctors will prescribe acyclovir ointment. But research shows that Mother Nature may have a more gentle solution. In fact, some medical doctors and honey proponents believe honey with its anti-inflammatory and healing properties works better than drugs for herpes—and it's natural, available without a doctor's okay, and cheap in comparison.

27 HOARSENESS (Get rid of the frog): Sores in the private parts or a raspy voice that everyone can hear—what is worse? Welcome to the sound of a voice that has rough notes. The most common causes are acute laryngitis to a cold, flu, or irritation linked to using your voice too much. Other less common and less serious links can be to allergies or sinusitis.

What Honey Rx to Use: Try a cup of hot tea (I recommend chamomile) with 1 tablespoon honey and 1 teaspoon fresh lemon juice. Repeat as needed. Combine this natural honey cure with drinking water. Turn on the humidifier (squeaky clean to prevent bacteria) if you live in a region with low humidity, like I do, and try to talk less rather than more.

Why You'll Bee Happy: While show hosts have told me my voice is "soothing," I give due credit to this honey cure, which coats the throat. Chamomile relaxes me and I've noticed that if you're in a comfort zone your voice will sound less raspy, too. Honey-lemon lozenges have helped me give a smoother performance and also soothe the itchy pain of overworked pipes.

28 HOT FLASHES (Run for the cool hive): A scratchy voice isn't fun, but hot flashes (yes, I experienced my share) aren't a tropical vacation, either, but can feel like one without making travel plans. One time at a Barnes & Noble book signing in Reno, Nevada, out of nowhere a hot flash paid me a visit. My face turned bright red. It was unsettling. I've learned triggers can include stress, heat, and hot beverages.

What Honey Rx to Use: Take 1 teaspoon of honey and pair it with iced tea, preferably chamomile or green.

Why You'll Bee Happy: A cold drink will refresh you and keep hot flashes at bay. Green tea is touted by Japanese women, who do not experience hot flashes like we American women do. And honey has a calming effect that will help get rid of that invasive warm rush, sooner rather than later.

29 IMMUNE SYSTEM BOOST (Get a daily immunity boost): Hot flashes come and go, as does a fever that may signal you that your immunity is down and a cold or flu is coming on. Did you know that your body is ready to go to war? In fact, it's on alert from the time you're born until the day you die. The enemies are viral and bacterial invaders that attack your health. Although you may not be aware of a potential battle going on, there are things you can do to stay healthy and keep the peace.

The answer lies in the immune system. The immune system—that is, your body's defense system, made up of billions of white blood cells or "warriors" that are ready to destroy potential enemies—can protect you against illness, including a cold, flu, bronchitis, and pneumonia, if it's fed the right superfoods.

What Honey Rx To Use: Put a teaspoon of medicinal honey in a cup of immunity-boosting tea for a double effect.

Why You'll Bee Happy: Enter honey with its antibacterial effects. "Honey can stimulate B-lymphocytes and T-lymphocytes to multiply, thus boosting the immune system," says *Honey: The Gourmet Medicine* author Joe Traynor.

30 INFERTILITY (Up your pregnancy odds): As a part-time phone psychic advisor who uses her intuitive gift, I often field calls from women who want to know when or if they will be with child. Sometimes I pick up the energy that there may be a need to nudge nature and recommend seeing their doctor to get the help they may need. However, there are folk remedies that also should be considered if you or someone you know needs a bit of a fertility boost.

What Honey Rx to Use: Eat royal jelly. Follow the instructions on the label for how much and how often you should indulge in the "food of royalty." It can be taken straight or in a smoothie. It's available at health-food stores.

Why You'll Bee Happy: Royal jelly is the stuff that a queen bee indulges in, and her fertility record is off the charts. This pricey bee product is chock-full of good-for-you essential minerals, B-complex vitamins, proteins, amino acids, collagen, essential fatty acids, and more nutrients. Sarah Ferguson ("Fergie") was noted to eat royal jelly while she was trying to become pregnant.[10]

31 **INSECT BITES (Take the itch away):** Getting pregnant can be a surprise, as can getting bit by an insect. The skin can become red and inflamed. Worse, if you're bit you'll want the pain to go away STAT. Honey may come to the rescue. Just ask me. I was bitten by a spider one winter. My cheekbone was painful and red. If I had known that there was a natural remedy to keep the swelling at bay I would have used it in between icing the area.

  What Honey Rx to Use: Put a light dressing of manuka honey on the bite(s) a few times per day.

  Why You'll Bee Happy: Medicinal honey, such as manuka, "has anti-inflammatory properties independent of its properties that combat bacterial infection. Inflammation has been reduced by honey when there were no infections involved," says former beekeeper Traynor. So, if you use honey and experience the inflammation diminishing from a painful insect bite, you won't be complaining.

32 **INSOMNIA (Find sweet dreams):** Getting bit hurts, but not getting adequate shut-eye can have long-term hurtful effects, too. Ever hit the hay and discover that when your eyes shut they open up again? You toss and turn or even turn on the tube. The clock is a barometer of your lack of

shut-eye. Counting sheep, thinking of pleasant thoughts—nothing seems to help you fall asleep and enter Slumberland.

What Honey Rx to Use: To try it, just take 1 or 2 teaspoons of your favorite honey, especially before going to bed. Want a double-duty potion? Try sipping a cup of hot 2 percent low-fat milk with a dash of cinnamon. The tryptophan in milk will help to calm you.

Why You'll Bee Happy: So, can honey help you to doze off? Yes, it can. It's magic trick, according to *The Honey Revolution* author Ron Fessenden, M.D., providing needed glycogen to the liver so the brain doesn't go in search of extra fuel in the early A.M. hours when you should be in Dreamland. "Consuming honey before bedtime also reduces the release of adrenaline, a catecholamine that raises blood pressure and heart rate," adds the honey guru.

33 **INTERSTITIAL CYSTITIS (Relieve the symptoms):** If anything can keep you from sleeping at night, it's a bout of cystitis (inflammation of the bladder, which causes the urge to urinate)—a problem for both women and men. Flare-ups can happen and can be annoying and enough to make you run, not walk, to a urologist. There are trigger foods, often high in acidity, that can trigger a bout of interstitial cystitis (IC), which is a chronic inflammation of the bladder. The good news is, honey is not a troublemaker, despite its acidity levels.

What Honey Rx to Use: Opt for a cup of chamomile tea (black tea can irritate the bladder) with a teaspoon of honey. If you have any problems, consider honey uses, including candles and cosmetics, that can be calming to you mentally and spiritually during a flare-up.

Why You'll Bee Happy: Jill H. Osborne, founder of the International Cystitis Network (ICN), says, "We've never had a complaint about honey triggering an IC flare." But she cautions IC survivors to stay clear of artificial sugars (which may trigger bladder discomfort), so sweet honey (or regular sugar) is the preferred sweetener of choice.

34 LACKLUSTER LIBIDO (Finding your groove, again): Speaking of woes below the belt, at any age your sex drive may wax and wane due to stress, hormones, work, kids, poor communication, or maybe you're just not that into him or her. Can honey give you a nudge to up your sex drive? Yes and no. As I have said before, I do not believe one superfood—even honey—can change your life, especially if your lifestyle is wreaking havoc on your body and mind. It's got to be a combo package. So, if you incorporate honey into your diet regime and eat healthy foods, exercise, are destressed, aren't overworked, send the kids to Happyland, communicate with you-know-who, and cope with out-of-whack hormones, yes, honey may help you feel frisky.

What Honey Rx to Use: Incorporate a small amount of royal jelly into your diet (in such foods as smoothies and cereal). The recommended use: 1 or 2 grams per day, notes Annie's Apitherapy. Follow instructions on the product label and consult with your health practitioner before you try this product from the hive, because bee products may cause an allergic reaction in some people.

Why You'll Bee Happy: Royal jelly, fit for a queen bee, may be helpful in the stress department, stave off symptoms of PMS (think cravings, crankies, and cramps), and lessen female and male menopause woes, such as fatigue and impotence, according to Annie's Apitherapy in Ontario, Canada.

If your libido makes a comeback you'll feel like a fertile queen or drone honey bee. Lovemaking does have plenty of virtues, boosting self-esteem, calming you, burning calories, promoting intimacy, improving sleep, and adding years to your life span, and it is pleasurable to feel connected to another human. That's right; making love is like finding your groove again.

Honey Love

She's as sweet as tupelo honey . . .
—Van Morrison, "Tupelo Honey"

Speaking of aphrodisiacs, honey and lovemaking have gone together like the birds and the bees since biblical times. Although less attention is paid to honey today as a libido enhancer, it was high on the list of aphrodisiac foods for the ancients, especially in Greece and Rome.

Did you know . . . honey, a timeless aphrodisiac, is included in the list of "foods for love"? Its name is used as an endearment, from "Honey Pie" to "My Honey." The word "honeymoon" was coined in ancient Europe because newlyweds derived their amatory stamina from drinking mead—a wine made from honey—during the first month of married life. Because honey is easily digested and has been absorbed as a super energy source for athletes since the ancient Olympics, think of the possibilities it holds for enhancing the sex drive when you are tired and tempted to mumble those three little words: "Not tonight, honey."

And honey's sex virtues, for both bees and humans, have been timeless. In Turkey, men believe honey can rev up the sex drive and Turkish women claim it recharges their sex appeal. The use of honey is also touted in classic books, including the *Kama Sutra*, an Indian work on sex, and *The Perfumed Garden*. What's more, the honey bee has an odd sex life. While workers are not sexual, a virgin queen bee mates with from six to more than a dozen drones in flight—a onetime ordeal; the drones are used for fertility and go to bee heaven shortly after. Others are pushed out of the hive come winter.

During my road adventures (like a virgin queen), I sipped and shared hot tea and honey with more than one man—but similar to drones, I was too restless to settle down in one place. Tea and honey were part of the romantic interludes. The tea (chamomile and green) had a calming effect for me, and the mild honey flavor with its instant fuel energized us both. As a result, intimate chat ended up in lingering pillow talk with everlasting memories that I cherish.

Honey Bee Sex Secrets

Energizing bee food, like honey, provides a quick energetic boost that can give both men and women the oomph to say, "Yes, tonight, honey," because they'll have a pick-me-up that works to make them feel in the mood for pleasuring, which takes physical stamina.

Erotic edibles can ignite the libido because of the sensory sensations. The sight of golden sweet and sticky honey matched with erotic foods, such as figs, dark chocolate, and juicy strawberries, can lead to spontaneous and uninhibited lovemaking.

Flower power can link honey and sex, because of honey's connection to aphrodisiac-type flowers—jasmine and orchids—with fragrant scents and shapes that lead to both romantic images and innuendo of a woman's genitals and virginity.

Raw Honey is believed to be a sexual aphrodisiac, since it contains substances such as zinc and vitamins B and E—the sexy nutrients that revitalize sex drive.

Sugar, like honey, is nature's helper that can help you to eat fewer high-fat foods and more low-fat, naturally sweet nutrient-dense fruits, vegetables, and whole grains that enhance heart health and blood flow to private parts for both men and women.

Honey has been a sweet ingredient with a sexual meaning—combined with other love foods—in lovers' recipes. These sexy foods can rekindle carnal desire. Sweet honey and romance go together like juicy strawberries and decadent dark chocolate, as you'll see in this recipe fit for a virgin bee, drone, or human ready for love.

Strawberry Chocolate Tart

❖ ❖ ❖

1⅔ cups slivered almonds
¼ cup butter or margarine, cut into pieces
3 tablespoons sugar
1 egg yolk
½ cup honey

½ cup unsweetened cocoa powder
1 teaspoon grated orange peel
2 teaspoons warm water
1 pint strawberries, hulled and sliced

Place toasted almonds in food processor with metal blade in place; process until finely ground. Add margarine, sugar and egg yolk; process until dough forms a ball. Chill 1 hour. Spray 9-inch tart pan (with removable bottom) generously with nonstick cooking spray. Press dough into bottom and up sides of tart pan. Dough will be sticky. Bake at 350°F degrees for 12 to 15 minutes, until shell is golden brown. Remove from oven and cool. In small bowl, whisk together honey, cocoa powder, orange peel and 2 teaspoons warm water. To assemble tart, spread chocolate filling into cooled tart shell. Arrange sliced strawberries in overlapping rings to cover. Refrigerate until ready to serve. Makes 8 servings.

(*Source:* National Honey Board.)

35 MORNING SICKNESS (Pamper your stomach):
Remember the saying: "First comes love, and
then comes marriage and then a baby carriage."
During pregnancy more than half of women will
cope with the trials and tribulations of an upset
tummy, usually during the first trimester. While
anticipating a new birth is a positive thing, reaching for crackers and hoping the queasies will fly
away like a honey bee is not a walk in the park, although that may be where a mom-to-be wishes
she could flee during a bout of nausea.

What Honey Rx to Use: Make a concoction by
putting 1 teaspoon of ginger root into 1 cup of
boiling water and simmering it for 10 minutes.
Strain and add lemon and honey to taste. Or
steep a bag in 1 cup of boiling water for a few
minutes.

Why You'll Bee Happy: Both ginger and honey
are touted to be a soothing natural medicine for
the stomach and intestines, relieving nausea. I
haven't given birth to a child, but I have experienced an upset stomach, especially if my furry
children were having tummy woes—I get upset
and get sympathy pains. The ginger honey tea
remedy calms me and can help calm a jumpy
stomach—helping me to be a better mom.

36 MUSCLE CRAMPS (Shake that sharp pain): Feeling queasy can wreak havoc on you, but a cramp
that hits for no reason, whether it be in a foot, a
leg, or even your stomach, can be enough to
make you holler, "Enough!" and pray for a cure
that works to work out that cramp.

What Honey Rx to Use: Drs. Patricia and Paul
Bragg advise taking 2 teaspoons apple cider vine-

gar and 1 teaspoon honey in a glass of distilled water three times per day.[11]

Why You'll Bee Happy: This folk remedy may work by allowing the precipitated acid crystals in your circulatory system to enter into a solution and pass out of the body. And if that doesn't do the trick, honey is a known muscle relaxant, so you've got two healing foods working together to work that cramp out of your life.[12]

37 PMS (Swat hormonal woes): Yes, menopausal years come with a mixed bag of monsters, but premenstrual syndrome isn't a bag of goodies, either. Ugh. I recall the scourge of PMS woes. Symptoms vary, but common complaints include cramps and chocolate cravings. Years ago, you weren't supposed to do the sugar dance, even if you craved to toss the cat and mate out the door, eat a carton of double chocolate-chip ice cream, and go to bed until the next century. When your out-of-whack hormones such as progesterone and estrogen wreak havoc on your well-being during PMSing, adding magnesium (a nutrient that can calm the nervous system)-rich dark honey can help soothe those frazzled nerves. That means less crankies.

What Honey Rx to Use: Try a spoonful of honey and a cup of chamomile tea.

Why You'll Bee Happy: Both sweet honey and tea will help you chill. Also, honey will help to give you an energy boost that can give you the desire to exercise or make love, and either activity can induce endorphins, which can reduce painful cramps and relax your nerves.

38 PREGNANCY (Control your blood pressure):
Speaking of PMS and hormones . . . some women
have a hard time with unwanted health problems
during their pregnant months, a challenging pe-
riod. I have had more than one friend who bat-
tled with high blood pressure, stress, and weight
gain during pregnancy.

What Honey Rx to Use: A fix of raw honey two or
three times daily. Use in a cup of herbal tea
and/or solo.

Why You'll Bee Happy: Honey has a calming effect on the nervous system, which in turn can
lower blood pressure and calm daily stressors.
Personally, one day I measured my blood pressure and it was higher than what it usually is. I ate
a teaspoon of creamed honey and waited 10 minutes. I took my blood pressure again and it was
below my normal reading. And I didn't have any
desire to turn to anxiety eating or comfort food,
which can pack on unwanted pounds.

39 SCARS (Minimize the effects): Scars often come
with the aftermath of a pregnancy or a cut, punc-
ture, or wound. Several years ago, my dog Simon
jumped up on the bed I was on and in his puppy
excitement scratched my face underneath the
nose. It was a semi-deep laceration but didn't re-
quire stitches. I asked the nurse if it would scar
and she didn't answer me. As I, and perhaps you,
too, know, preventing scarred tissue is a challenge. Some honey proponents believe honey
may minimize scarring if used on a wound.

What Honey Rx to Use: Apply a small amount of
honey, preferably manuka, to a wound with cotton

before applying a bandage (or purchase manuka bandages for convenience).

Why You'll Bee Happy: It is a known fact that when honey is exposed to air it acts like a moisture magnet. This action, in turn, may be helpful in lessening scarring by keeping the skin moist during the process of the formation of new, improved tissue. There are pricey commercial anti-scarring salves available, but with honey's reputation for healing skin, it's worth a go for both two-leggers and four-leggers.

40 **SEASONAL AFFECTIVE DISORDER (Uplift your spirits):** Scars are a burden, but so are seasonal hang-ups. If it's January or February and you find yourself with unwanted winter body fat, irritable, and fed up with the shorter days, colder nights, and lack of sunshine and warmth, you may be suffering from Seasonal Affective Disorder (SAD), coined by Dr. Norman Rosenthal, who endured the telltale symptoms. Sufferers know too well that low moods, weight gain, and anxiety, especially in the winter months, are part of the package. But don't despair, because honey can be helpful.

What Honey Rx to Use: Try a cup of hot tea with milk and honey. Repeat as needed. Or opt for a teaspoon of creamed or liquid honey and exercise immediately after.

Why You'll Bee Happy: People with SAD often have low levels of serotonin (a compound found in honey and milk), a brain chemical believed to be involved in modulating mood and appetite. By eating tryptophan-rich foods such as milk sweetened with honey you can boost levels of serotonin.

41 SINUSITIS (Do away with sinus misery): In the winter SAD can be dreadful, but in fall, winter, spring, and summer people with sinus woes can be miserable, too. We're talking headache, sneezing, congestion, and more. Cold weather compounded with lack of humidity and central house heating (or indoor air-conditioning in hot weather) can exacerbate your symptoms.

What Honey Rx to Use: Opt for a teaspoon of honey, three times a day, during the time you feel a bout of sinusitis on its way. Or take one chew of honeycomb every hour for four to six hours. Chew each amount for 15 minutes and discard what remains in your mouth.[13]

Why You'll Bee Happy: "When inflammation of one or more of the sinuses appears, it develops on an alkaline-urine-reaction background. When honeycomb is chewed the urine reaction is shifted from alkaline to acid, showing how quickly honeycomb brings about a change in body chemistry," explains folk medicine doctor D. C. Jarvis.[14]

42 SKIN DRYNESS (Take care of your skin): Not only do I face sinus problems, but moisturizing skin with an SPF (sun protection factor) is a must, especially in high altitude. The wintertime is harsh, thanks to the heater being on 24/7, and since I swim year-round, chlorine doesn't help. It can be drying to your hands and feet. Not to forget the chances of getting athlete's foot from the cement around the pools. And the sun, wherever you are, can be hard on your skin, too. What's more, when I bring wood into the house to make a fire I've cut my hands more than once, not to forget falling on snow-covered ground— more cuts and scrapes.

What Honey Rx to Use: Wash hands with manuka honey soap and lather well. Using a lot of friction helps to get rid of dead skin and germs. Rinse thoroughly and dry.

Why You'll Bee Happy: Manuka honey helps the skin absorb and retain moisture. Manuka honey also contains vitamins, amino acids, and antioxidants that are good for the skin. Manuka soap can be helpful for different uses, including moisturizing dry skin, cleaning infected wounds, cleaning acne and eczema, removing facial makeup, treating athlete's foot, reducing the appearance of wrinkles, and killing bacteria on the surface of the skin that cause infections. (I've used a variety of honey soaps—and have enjoyed them all. My favorite is Honeymark Manuka Honey Soap. It's handmade (UMF 16+) and from New Zealand.)

43 SLUGGISH SPORTS PERFORMANCE (Farewell to lack of energy): If you've got a sinus infection, you won't feel like running a marathon or doing much of anything that requires physical exertion. As a kid, I was a competitive swimmer. While I was busy coping with butterflies in my stomach before performing in front of a crowd, it was a sweet fix that my dad gave to me. A candy bar was the fuel of choice before swimming the backstroke in that 25-yard swimming pool. These days, after I swim the breaststroke I turn to a small piece of chocolate to curb my big appetite, and this way I stave off the urge to overeat and gaining unwanted weight.

What Honey Rx to Use: A chocolate candy bar, or honey, will do the trick before you perform a physical race or task. A bonus tip: Drink a cup of brewed coffee before your physical performance.

Why You'll Bee Happy: Athletes are all too familiar with the energetic buzz linked to the properties of quality sweets. Not only does it enhance energy, but it also curbs distracting hunger pangs before they participate in a physical event. And yes, brewed coffee contains caffeine (approximately 85 milligrams per 8-ounce mug), much more than chocolate (1 ounce of semi-sweet dark chocolate contains about 20 milligrams of caffeine). I can vouch that coffee and honey can boost endurance and performance. Remember, moderation.

Honey Is an Athlete's Team Player

Staying on the top of your game in exercise takes more than a spoonful of energizing honey, providing a carbohydrate content of 17 grams. But honey, the natural energizer, can work for your working muscles, since carbs are the main fuel the body uses for energy. In Nutrition 101 students are taught that carbs are essential in the diet to help maintain muscle glycogen—stored carbs—which are the most important fuel source for athletes to help them keep going.

Honey Power

Honey is an ideal athletic aid for athletes and everyday people who get physical and want to stay fit.

Preexercise: Sports nutritionists, past and present, have advised and do advise eating carbs before an athletic activity for an energy boost. Pure honey steps up to the plate when eaten before a workout or other activity. How? How does it do it? Simply put, honey is released into the system at a steady rate throughout physical activity.

During exercise: Turning to honey during a workout helps your muscles stay nourished longer and puts off fatigue.

Postexercise: Researchers have shown that a combo of carbs and protein after physical activity (within 30 minutes) can refuel and delay the onset of muscle soreness. What's more, carb-protein combos can help keep your blood-sugar levels steady after exercise.

Power up with honey: Staying hydrated is important for anyone who gets physical. Add honey to a bottle of water for an energy re-jump-start during your next workout; try mixing peanut butter and honey, or honey and light cream cheese, as a dip for fresh fruits or vegetables. Peanut butter and honey sandwiches on wholewheat bread will give you a high-energy bite and you'll get carbs, protein, and fat. Honey is a convenient, on-the-go source of energy; take it with you for athletic events to help power up and recharge your energy.

(*Source:* National Honey Board.)

44 TENSION (Escape tense times): If you've got an energetic buzz, you may want to flee tense times due to pressure on the job, at-home conflicts with family, friends or neighbors, or events that cannot be controlled. The key to chilling is learning how to go with the flow—and finding natural ways to help you deal.

What Honey Rx to Use: Try 1 teaspoon of honey in a glass of fresh fruit juice, such as orange, grapefruit, prune, or cranberry, all rich in heart-healthy potassium, your blood pressure's best friend.

Why You'll Bee Happy: If you include fresh juices teamed with honeys in your day-to-day diet regime, you'll be getting antistress B and C vitamins, and these good-for-you nutrients can help you to stay cool and calm during the roller-coaster times that we all face one time or another. It's the combination of nature's remedies, like these, that can work on those nerves when tension rises and you need a little help from the honey bee's gifts.

45 **THROAT SOOTHER (Take the sting away):** Tension is a drag, but a sore throat can drag you down, too, where you don't feel like walking or talking. Honey has been used as a home cure for centuries to help soothe one of the symptoms associated with a common cold—namely, a killer sore throat. According to the American Association of Family Physicians, many things can cause a sore throat, including infections with viruses, such as colds and flu; sinus drainage; and allergies.

What Honey Rx to Use: For relief of symptoms, take a spoonful of your buckwheat honey, as often as you need, to relieve irritation. In between, sip a cup of tea with honey. Also, try pure honeycomb and honey sticks. Don't forget all-natural honey-lemon lozenges, which also coat the throat for quick relief.

Why You'll Bee Happy: Let me count the ways. One, honey will coat your sore throat, the symptom of a cause. Two, the antibacterial and anti-inflammatory properties will help heal the culprit causing your pain.

46 TICS AND TWITCHES (Dodge muscle quirks):

Sore throat and a twitching muscle can both be irritating. I recall one day my left eyelid twitched off and on for about two hours. There was no reason—and not only was it annoying, but I was clueless to why it happened also.

What Honey Rx to Use: Take 1 teaspoon of honey and chill, whether you are meditating or exercising.

Why You'll Bee Happy: My choice of cures to chase away that odd eye twitch was taking a teaspoon of honey (I chose an apricot crème) and hitting the swimming pool. After about 30 minutes of lap swimming the eye twitch was history. "Honey contains acetylcholine, which acts as a chemical transmitter of nerve impulses," explains Traynor. So, I believe the combination of taking honey and destressing is the cure for minor tics and twitches with an unknown cause.

47 WAIST WHITTLER (Blast belly fat): Twitches to

tummy bulge . . . if you have a bulging tummy, you'd probably consider a twitch easier to get rid of. But wait; there are things you can do to get a flatter tummy. With the right diet and exercise, anyone can tame the bulge and have a young-looking, flatter stomach. And versatile honey can help shrink your tummy.

What Honey Rx to Use: Both morning and night, drink an 8-ounce glass or mug of tea (dandelion or parsley boasts diuretic effects), with a teaspoon of honey and a teaspoon of apple cider vinegar. Team this potion with grazing and watching your fat and sugar intake.

Why You'll Bee Happy: Honey and apple cider vinegar contain the bloat-busting mineral potassium, as does produce. But eating smaller, more frequent meals is also key to getting a trimmer waist and keeping your metabolism revved up. Plus, cutting down on high-fat refined carbs, such as candy bars and cookies, will help you to minimize belly fat, too. Turning to honey will help you to eat fewer sugary treats and enjoy a flatter stomach.

48 WOUNDS (Heal Wounds): Once you've got a flat stomach, what do you do if you stub your toe or cut your finger? Honey is believed by scientists, such as Dr. Peter Molan (refer to chapter 3), to be one of the nature's most powerful wound dressings, which really works. As I've noted many times already, honey has antibacterial properties. But that's not all. . . .

What Honey Rx to Use: Try manuka honey, available in many forms. It's available online in lotions, creams, and bandages. Apply as directed.

Why You'll Bee Happy: Honey can numb pain. It is osmotic and attracts water. Since bacteria are mostly made of water, they are sucked dry in the presence of honey. Bacteria are further inhibited by honey because the golden liquid produces hydrogen peroxide and is acidic (like vinegar). Honey activates the immune response by providing glucose for the white blood cells. It speeds up the healing process. It creates a moist environment by drawing serum up through the skin tissues that helps "moist scab" formation.

What's more, honey also reduces inflammation, helps shed dead tissue, and stimulates the development of new blood cells. Honey's antiseptic qualities also help prevent infections from moving to other wounds. On a personal note, I did cut my toe on the deck. I turned to manuka honey despite my younger brother's mocking my choice of remedy. Two days later, the once-unsightly wound was nearly healed.

49 WRINKLE AND GRAVITY FIGHTER (Nourish aging skin): Wounds can heal with the help of honey, and honey can also smooth your skin. Although antioxidant skin nutrients—found in honey—are essential to maintaining antiaging skin, other things play a role, too. During your forties, oil glands are less active, which means moisturizing is more important. Skin is not as firm in your fifties, due to the breakdown of collagen, which gives skin its elasticity. The solution is more moisture, which gives it elasticity.

What Honey Rx to Use: Eat vitamin E food sources, which include wheat germ, almonds, sunflower seeds, and legumes, with honey.

Why You'll Bee Happy: Antioxidant skin nutrients are essential to maintaining antiaging skin.

Also, using honey moisturizers (refer to chapter 13) can provide more moisture—a must-have for smoother skin. At every age, dermatologists stress using sunscreen daily with an SPF at all times when outdoors; wearing sunglasses to protect your eyes from harmful ultraviolet rays and to stave off squinting that worsens crow's-feet; getting as much sleep as you can (honey can help here); and exercising regularly to boost circulation, which will improve skin texture and tone (energizing honey will give you that urge to go do it).

50 **UNIVERSAL EMERGENCY AID (Opt for an all-purpose worker):** A sore throat can hurt, but an untimely event, such as a blizzard, earthquake, hurricane, or wildfire, is much worse. Imagine grabbing a few of your belongings, including a first-aid kid, and getting the heck out of Dodge. Or staying put. Either way, having honey on hand in time of disaster can be a godsend if you must endure a cut, or stomachache, need an energetic boost, or even suffer from dry skin.

What Honey Rx to Use: Put a basic honey, such as clover or alfalfa, *and* medicinal manuka honey into sealed plastic containers and store these honey products with your emergency supplies.

Why You'll Bee Happy: If you experience a major quake, hurricane, tornado, or flood or are stuck in a car during a snowstorm, having honey can help, from keeping a cut from getting infected to soothing frazzled nerves. During a natural or man-made disaster, honey just may be the essential lifesaver that you'll be glad you packed away for emergency preparedness. Eating honey can help boost the immune system, which is vital during a stressful event, and lower the risk of heart disease (yes, it calms, and that can prevent your blood pressure from skyrocketing). Also, honey—in a variety of forms—can help relieve insomnia (often a problem after a traumatic happening) as well as give you energy when you're feeling tired and challenged. During WW II soldiers had honey, and back in the ancient times Greek and Roman warriors used honey for cuts and wounds. It is the ultimate cure-all in time of need and should be part of your first-aid kid in the home, office, and car.

UN-BEE-LIEVABLE HEALING HINTS TO CATCH

If the following chart doesn't specify which variety of honey to use, go ahead and use your own preference: all-natural, raw honey, dark varietals are recommended for best results.

Ailment or Other Purpose	Form of Honey	What It May Do
Acne	Honey facial with other superfoods	Clear your skin
Allergies	Alfalfa honey	Relieve sneezing and congestion
Anemia	Honey	Boost red blood cells

Ailment or Other Purpose	Form of Honey	What It May Do
Anxiety	Honey and tea	Soothe frazzled nerves
Bad breath	Honey	Freshen mouth
Bedsores	Honey	Aid in healing
Bed-wetting	Honey	Relax nervous system
Blahs	Honey	Boost feel-good endorphins
Bone loss	Honey and yogurt	Strengthen bones
Burns	Manuka honey	Soothe smarting and inflammation
Cavities	Honey	Aid in healthier teeth
Colds/flus	Cranberry, wild-flower or acacia	Speed recovery
Cold sores	Honey	Help healing
Constipation	Honey	Aid in regularity
Cough	Honey	Soothe tickle

Ailment or Other Purpose	Form of Honey	What It May Do
Depression	Honey	Uplift spirit
Detoxifcation	Chestnut honey	Cleanse body toxins
Diarrhea	Honey	Help regulation
Digestive problems	Honey	Soothe stomach upset
Energy drain	Honey	Boost energy levels
Eye health	Honey	Protect vision
Fibromyalgia	Honey	Lessen aches and pains
Gallstones	Honey	Prevent gallstones
Hangover	Honey	Speed recovery
Headache	Acacia honey	Relieve pain
Heartburn	Honey	Alleviate the burn
Herpes	Honey	Aid in healing

Ailment or Other Purpose	Form of Honey	What It May Do
Hoarseness	Honey	Soothe raspy voice
Hot flashes	Honey	Maintain normal temperature
Immune system boost	Honey	Maintain strong immunity
Infertility	Honey	Enhance fertility
Insect bites	Honey	Heal inflammation
Insomnia	Honey	Aid relaxation and sleep
Interstitial cystitus	Honey	Relax and soothe muscles
Lackluster libido	Honey	Rev up sex drive, energize, calm, and enhance stamina
Morning sickness	Honey	Help queasiness
Muscle cramps	Honey	Relax nervous system

Ailment or Other Purpose	Form of Honey	What It May Do
PMS	Honey	Lessen cramps and crankies
Pregnancy	Honey	Lower high blood pressure
Scars	Manuka honey	Heal scar tissue
Seasonal Affective Disorder	Honey	Boost mood and energy and lessen simple carb cravings
Sinusitus	Honeycomb	Relieve stuffed-up nasal passages
Skin dryness	Manuka	Help dry skin
Sluggish sports performance	Honey bar	Energize and increase stamina
Tension	Honey	Calm nervous system
Throat soother	Honey	Soothe the throat
Tics and twitches	Honey	Calm nervous impulses

Ailment or Other Purpose	Form of Honey	What It May Do
Universal emergency	Honey	Act as cure-all aid
Waist whittler	Honey	Help get rid of belly fat
Wounds	Manuka honey	Heal
Wrinkle and fighter	Honey	Aid in smoothing skin

In chapter 12, "Honeymania: Honey for the Household," you'll find out about the sweet buzz that has stuck around for centuries thanks to its versatile, natural uses in the home.

PART 7

FUTURE HONEY

Honeymania: Honey for the Household

When you shoot an arrow of truth, dip its point in honey.

—Arab proverb[1]

Like a field bee making a beeline to its colony, I returned home to San Jose, a region still plentiful in corn fields, lemon and apple trees, and flower gardens. My life included the three of us: one motocross racer; my dog, Stone Fox; and me. We found a garden apartment in the South Bay.

A typical night before a race, I'd be in the kitchen of our garden apartment. Busy as a worker bee, I'd create peanut butter honey balls. In a bowl I'd mix up peanut butter, raisins, nuts, and honey to hold it all together like honeycomb. On our drives to different races, we both enjoyed the honey balls for energy and a feel-good boost.

The summer before our domesticated San Jose lifestyle, we camped outdoors like wild bees in Sonora, gold miner's country. Again, I was amid nature with the Tuolumne River, trees, and flowers—a honey bee's paradise. I remember making sun tea laced with honey. A local woman watched me working, sunning, and swimming in the river with my lab. She called out to us, "Life is short and you'll remember days like this!" Today, her words ring true. I can envision the freedom of traveling from place to place like a honey bee.

In this chapter, I will show you that while honey is used as a food, it's also making a splash in the United States and around the world for other reasons. There's the amazing world of honey and how it's used in amazing ways. The nectar of the gods is "in" and appreciated both indoors and in the great outdoors, wherever your honey bee spirit guides you.

THE HONEY CRAZE

The National Honey Board's recent survey shows that a pro-honey attitude is on the mark, sort of. More than 500 households, both men and women between the ages of 21 and 74, were contacted to find out about their honey attitude:

- 65 percent of households currently use and have honey in their home.
- 60 percent of respondents reported purchasing honey within the past year.
- One-quarter of the total number of respondents did not know that pure honey has no other ingredients. Those who believed there were ingredients added to honey expected to find syrups, sugars, and/or preservatives on the ingredient list.

- More than two-fifths of all households indicate they are willing to pay a premium of about 10 percent for whole-wheat bread, barbeque sauce, and breakfast cereal made with honey.
- For the total number of respondents, it was reported that honey was primarily used as a sweetener in beverages and / or as a spread on toast and thus was used most often at breakfast.

(*Source:* National Honey Board, 2009.)

WIDESPREAD HONEY APPEAL

While honey is a household name in the kitchen for people in the United States, it is praised for its edible uses around the globe, too. If traveling in another country, you'll find these honeys can be a fruitful experience (like tasting chocolate in foreign countries), as imports are sweet but not as fresh to the palate.

Honey Type	Country(ies) of Origin
Acacia	Eastern Europe (Hungary, Romania, Bulgaria)
Apple blossom	UK
Borage	UK/New Zealand
Cherry blossom	UK
Clover	Canada / New Zealand
Eucalyptus	Australia

Honey Type	Country(ies) of Origin
Hawthorn	UK
Lavender	France/Spain
Leatherwood	Tasmania
Lime blossom	China/UK/Poland
Orange blossom	Spain/Mexico
Rosemary	France/Spain
Strawberry clover	Australia
Wild thyme	Greece/New Zealand/France/Spain
Sunflower	France/Spain

(*Source:* The Honey Association.)

BEESWAX IN YOUR HIVE

Welcome to the world of beeswax, another gift of the honey bee. Before I entered Honeyland, I was clueless to using this honey product in my home. I've discovered that it is a common household item that is used for lots of essential needs. We're talking candles, soaps, and furniture polishes.

Once you try beeswax candles, honey soap, and home-made beeswax furniture polish it's going to be a task to go back to whatever it was that you were using before. If beeswax items make it into your home, they will be a much-appreciated staple.

CANDLES—A BEE-AUTIFUL GIFT

I love the warmth and ambiance candles create in my home. The glow of candles makes each room in your home more inviting. In the kitchen, a scented candle provides a nice effect when you're cooking and baking. When you are serving a meal at any time of the day, candles in the dining room or living room can make the occasion more special and comforting. Moving on into the bathroom, we all know candles can provide a relaxing spa-type experience. And from the living room to the bedroom, from dusk to late night, flickering candles are more soothing and romantic than a bright light.

In ancient Egypt, tombs revealed carvings of candles. During the Middle Ages in Europe, only the wealthy could afford beeswax candles. In 1857, paraffin wax, stearin, and a wick were combined to create candles everyone could afford. Nowadays, beeswax is often used to make candles and beeswax candles are in many ways better than the popular paraffin candles—less costly but with a price to pay when it comes to your health and well-being. After all, the beeswax candles are 100 percent pure. What's more, they burn a clean, hot, and bright flame, are long lasting, create minimal smoke, and are nontoxic and nonallergenic. And that's not all. . . .

Dutchman's Gold's bee experts explain that beeswax is a natural wax—and immediately the word "natural" has got my attention. As they tell it, beeswax is secreted by the glands of honey bees as they do their work of producing and storing honey in the hive. Not only does beeswax have a natural scent—like the floral source from which the bees gather nectar—but when beeswax candles are burned they make negative ions that remove toxins and impurities from the air. Think philodendron plants and make room in your house for the natural candle, a gift to you from the honey bee and their people who make candles.

A Candlestick Maker's Beeswax Story

Ferdinand Knorr came to the United States in 1904 after fleeing from his native Poland and the Russian Czar. Tinkering in his machine shop and enjoying his hobby of beekeeping proved to be a successful combination. Fred produced an improved honeycomb for his bees and his famous candles soon followed . . . candles that were dripless, smokeless, and had a gentle scent.

The candles were developed in 1928 and initially sold to gift shops and a local inn.

The business took off like a forager bee and has been operated by his family since the mid 20th century.

Henry, Judy, and new owner Steve have made Knorr Candle Factory an ongoing success by using the finest materials and holding on to traditional manufacturing methods. Knorr's high quality dripless 100 percent beeswax candles with wicks are a welcome addition to homes in all fifty states and around the globe.

Speaking of locale, 160,000 bees must travel 150,000 miles collecting nectar to produce 60 pounds of honey that yield only 1 pound of beeswax.

A do-it-yourself candle-making kit with candle rolling instructions paid me a visit, thanks to Knorr's. I received all earth-tone colors from the Beeswax Candle Color Palette. At first, the instructions appeared challenging (I flunked the IQ test in grade school and the army test, too: it had lots of math and tool recognition). So, when I first saw the diagrams my thought was, *I'm out of here.* But then, it made sense. Diagram A shows how to roll one 8-inch candle; Diagram B shows how to roll two 4¼-inch candles, and Diagram C shows how to roll one jumbo 4¼-inch candle. But note, it's easy once you get the hang of it after a few tries, and easier than making candles from scratch over a hot stove. I'll save that project for a snow day.

THE ABCs OF BURNING BEESWAX CANDLES

Is there really a fine art to burning beeswax candles? Well, if you want to enjoy those beautiful tea lights, tapers, molds, and pillars, yes, there are some tips to help you get it right the first time.

- To ensure even-burning and dripless features, keep all beeswax candles away from drafts and ceiling fans.

- Do not leave burning candles unattended.

- Keep out of reach of children and companion animals. Remove any potential flammable material from the vicinity of candles.

- Pillar candles are more high maintenance than tapers. To keep pillars in tiptop shape, trim the wick when needed to 1/4 inch. Always put out the flame using a candle snuffer. Be sure the ember is out.

- When pillar candles are fully extinguished, pour off excess liquid wax into a nonflammable container. With a knife or sharp tool, trim outside edges on the top of the candle down to the height of the top wick.

(*Source:* Dutchman's Gold.)

SWEET HOLIDAYS, SWEET HONEY

As a kid raised Catholic I can remember honey played a role during the holidays in suburbia where I grew up. Even on Fridays (no meat) honey played a role with our glazed fish dinners. In the winter, on special days such as Valentine's Day, my mother would always make a dinner including honey-basted game hens, wild rice, green peas, and homemade biscuits paired with clover honey. During Easter, a honey-baked ham was a tradition in our home. And in the summer, on the Fourth of July, fried chicken and corn bread slathered with honey didn't get ignored at neighborhood block parties.

In the fall, birthdays in October were celebrated with tea and honey because this was the month that usually one of my siblings or I caught a cold or flu. Thanksgiving was a main event and a honey-glazed turkey was served on our dining room table. Once Christmas vacation rolled around and through the New Year's holiday, cookies—all types—were baked and often infused with honey. Honey was part of our household and made each holiday special. But I'm hardly alone in celebrating the golden nectar, and its ways differ from religion to religion.

HOLY HONEY

Take a look at other ways honey is used in households, be it as food or decorations for honoring different religions.

Religion	Uses
Buddhism	Honey is used in the festival of Madhu Purnima, observed in India and Bangladesh. Buddhists give honey to the monks in memory of the legend of a monkey bringing Buddha honey while he was making peace among his disciples in the wilderness.
Christianity/ Catholicism	Honey is used in beeswax candles. Religious candles are used for decoration and observance of holy holidays, including baptisms, confirmations, Christmas, and Easter, as well as altar candles.

Religion	Uses
Christianity/ Catholicism	Honey is used in grasshopper pie to remember John the Baptist, who, as a legend tells it, survived in the wild on a diet of locust and wild honey.
Hinduism	Honey is one of five elixirs of immortality. In temples honey is poured over deities in a ritual dubbed Madhu abhisheka.
Judaism	Honey is a symbol for the New Year, Rosh Hashanah. The tradition is apple slices dipped in honey.

Honey To-Do List: The week before your honey holiday invite friends and family; familiarize yourself with the traditional ceremony; buy special foods and items at online sites, which offer a wide variety; write out recipes and a menu; and purchase small honey-related gift items. The day of your holiday create a bee-autiful table setting and make the food.

BEESWAX WORKERS

Making your own all-natural beeswax polish seems easy enough, but I gravitated toward a ready-made product. The Original Bee's Wax Old World Formula Furniture Polish snagged my interest. This is dubbed as "America's Premier Furniture Polish since 1974" and has natural beeswax. I captured the magic of beeswax because of this polish's convenient-to-use aerosol form (visit their website: www.beeswaxpolish.com).

It lives up to the promise that it's the one furniture polish that "won't fingerprint; leaves no wax buildup; makes granite and marble acid resistant; needs no buffing; and enhances the true natural beauty of all wood." It's good to use on antiques, kitchen cabinets, wrought iron, porcelain, mirrors, marble, leather, glass, stainless steel, and more. In my Old Tahoe–style cabin with a Mediterranean charm, it made my antique dining room table with wrought iron shine. I fell in love with this beeswax furniture polish. But there are other choices if you want a DIY furniture polish or other household cleaners. . . .

Beeswax Polish

Beeswax furniture polish with its soft, satin shine is considered the ultimate in wood care. Note that there is very little difference between this formula and the formula for shoe polish.

4 ounces (weight) beeswax
2 tablespoons carnauba wax
2½ cups odorless turpentine or mineral spirits

Melt the waxes on high in a microwave or in a double boiler. Remove the waxes from the heat and stir in the turpentine or mineral spirits. Apply the polish with a clean cloth and rub in small circles. Turn the cloth as it becomes dirty. Allow the polish to dry, then buff with a clean cloth. If more than one coat is desired, wait two days between applications.

Copper Cleaner

42 parts soap flakes
42 parts vinegar, 5 percent to 7 percent acetic acid

2.4 parts beeswax
9.2 parts mineral oil
42 parts citric acid, USP crystals

Combine the soap and vinegar to make a paste. Melt the beeswax and mineral oil together in a microwave or double boiler. Stir in the soap mixture and the citric acid. Let the cleaner set overnight before using it. Apply the polish with a clean, damp cloth. Rinse the copper and wipe it dry with a clean cloth.

Spice Sachets

1½ oz. weight beeswax
1 cup applesauce
1½ cups ground cinnamon or a mixture of cinnamon, nutmeg, allspice, and cloves
Up to 1 teaspoon of essential oil from any of the spices may also be added.

Heat the wax and applesauce in a microwave or double boiler until the wax is melted. Stir in the ground spices. Knead the mixture until it is dough-like. Roll the dough into sheets and cut out forms or hand-form the dough into balls or beads. Place the forms on cardboard. They will harden in 3 or 4 days. The fragrance will last for years.

(*Source:* Courtesy of SoulShine Beeswax Candles; www.soulshinecandles@charter.net.)

HONEY SPILLS ON YOUR STUFF?

Honey is a household must-have, but what happens when you or the kids spill honey on that sofa, love seat, or chair? First, scrape honey off sooner rather than later rather instead of letting it dry. Next, use your favorite mild liquid soap diluted in a cup of cold water. Repeat as needed. Also, you can try a mixture of lemon, white vinegar, and water. Let dry and the honey mark should be history. The same treatment can work for garments. Again, act fast and chances are sweet honey will not sour your favorite things.

HEALTHY HONEY FENG SHUI TIPS

Welcome your sweet home to the art of honey-ized feng shui—the ancient Chinese art of placement. Its goal is to bring you peace and harmony. By putting stuff in the right spots in your kitchen and other rooms you can enhance the flow of positive energy and zap negative vibrations. The end result: good health, happiness—and even fortune. Read on—you, too, can enjoy a well-balanced hive that feels good from head to toe, with a touch of honey.

Use beeswax cleaners. It's time to clean your kitchen from top to bottom to be clean like a clean beehive. If you keep it eco-friendly it will provide you with better health and energy.

Declutter your honeys. Getting rid of things you don't use will up your energy. You will feel lighter with less kitchen baggage. I cleaned out my pantry and added a fresh box of baking soda to soak up odors. Then I tackled each honey jar and wiped each one, one by one (yes, they do last forever, but some packers recommend a two-year shelf life).

Clean the stovetop and oven. This was a chore, but it feels right to have the stovetop shine. Use vinegar and water. Trust me, this is a feel-good must-do before baking and cooking with honey.

Brighten up with lighting. You'll want to have sunny-type lighting, which can up your energy and is mood linked to good health. Go for full-spectrum lightbulbs. And, of course, remember honey can help boost your mood, too. The brighter the light, the better you can see which type of honey varietals to use.

Boost your mood with plants. To help wipe out pollutants in your kitchen—like beekeepers do with their colonies—fill your space with healthy, hardy, happy plants. Your best bet: philodendrons.

Bring on the water. Fish aquariums provide positive energy in the dining room, especially with a gentle filter.

Fish, fish, fish. I read that goldfish can bring you good luck and prosperity. In fact, nine is the lucky number (and so is eight). The colors? Gold and one black one. The fish are a pleasant, calming treat. Also, this is a good strategy, for when you cook and bake honey dishes the odds are better that they will turn out better.

Bring out the fresh fruit. Keep healthful seasonal fruits on display and ready to cut and pair with honeys. The feng shui gurus believe a full bowl may lead to a full life. Empty bowls with just a few pieces of fruit gone bad are not so good. And oranges? Nine is the lucky number. Put them in a wooden bowl and on the kitchen or dining room table. The bowl will be a sweet reminder to keep it filled and to keep getting your vitamin C each day teamed with antioxidant-rich honey.

Conceal knives and scissors. My father gave me a black and white marble knife block, cutting board, and rolling pin. I love it. But the knives are out of sight. I do use these for onions and garlic and to open a sealed jar of honey or a package of honeycomb. (My black cat Kerouac likes to chew on the black knife tops. Yes, black cats can and do bring good luck.)

Hang pots and pans. My cooking stuff is hanging on

the wall in a perfect hexagon arrangement—like a six-sided beehive. I'm thinking about getting one of those artsy-looking overhead pot-and-pan hangers (it would remind me of a honey bee in transit). If so, I will not, nor should you, hang it over a workplace, the area where honey recipes to live for are created. Not good energy, or so the feng shui wizards claim.

Hide the gadget honeys. Too many jars of honey can clutter up all that positive decluttering you did. Also, you want to keep honeys stored in a dark, cool place.

Hang wind chimes with crystals. If you don't have a colony (or more) so you can hear buzzing sounds, wind chimes may suffice. I brought one of mine in from the deck and put it over the kitchen windows. The one I chose is of a honey bee. Hanging chimes in the doorway to the kitchen or over the stove buzzes good energy.

A bonus tip: Purchase a honey bee calendar. It will provide you with inspiration when you use honey in your meals, and, of course, the dates of lunar cycles and seasons will remind you of what the honey bee is doing in your state.

FUN ART STUFF FOR ADULTS AND KIDS

Wax Crayons

Parts by weight:
2 parts beeswax
1 part talc
Pigment

Melt the wax in a microwave or small can placed in boiling water (a double boiler). Stir in the talc and dry artist's pigment or fresco colors. Pour the mixture into a lubricated aluminum foil mold. The crayon may be melted again and more pigment added until it is the exact color desired. Caution: These crayons should not be used by children because some pigments are not food safe.

Wax Pastels

Parts by weight:
1 part beeswax
1 part grated soap
Pigment

Melt the beeswax in a small can placed in boiling water. Add the grated soap and stir until the soap melts and the mixture is smooth. Color the mixture with dry artist's pigment or fresco colors. Pour into lubricated aluminum foil molds. After testing the crayon, it can be melted again and more pigment added. Caution: These crayons should not be used by children because some pigments are not food safe.

Wax Pastels for Children

Follow the directions above for "Wax Pastels" using concentrated food coloring as the pigment. The paste is sold with cake decorating supplies. The crayons are food safe and they blend well. Their color is almost as concentrated as the crayons made with the artist's pigment.

(*Source:* Courtesy of SoulShine Beeswax Candles; www.soulshinecandles@charter.net.)

Is Honey a Pet's Best Friend?

Like apple cider vinegar and olive oil, honey is rich in antioxidants and antibacterial properties—and has its place in the pet world, both internally and topically. Scientific research proves honey works to heal abscesses, burns, and surgical wounds. Manuka honey, available from Dechra Veterinary Products, is now being used by vets to treat wounds. It has been shown to fight more than 70 strains of bacteria found in wounds. But that's not all. . . .[2]

Not only can honey be used topically on animals, but honey is also used in some commercial pet treats and do-it-yourself recipes, too. Here is a sweet treat for four-legged companions.

Homemade Treats for Your Dog
Spicy Treat-Balls

❖ ❖ ❖

⅔ cup whole-wheat flour
⅓ cup white flour
½ cup bran
½ cup brewer's yeast
¼ cup wheat germ
½ teaspoon cinnamon
3 tablespoons honey
2 tablespoons corn oil
1 egg
⅓ cup milk

Preheat oven to 350°F. In a large bowl, combine dry ingredients. In a separate bowl, beat honey, corn oil, egg and milk. Gradually add mixture to dry ingredients to form a dough. Form into 1-inch balls and bake at 350°F on an ungreased cookie sheet for 15 minutes. Makes 18 balls. [For safety's sake, check with your veterinarian before you give Spicy Treat-Balls to your canine companion.]

(*Source:* Courtesy of PetPlace Veterinarians.)

Now that I've put versatile honey in the limelight and explained how to use it to make a happy home and maintain healthy kids and pets, take a look at how the ancient food of the gods—either solo or as an ingredient in ready-made beauty products and do-it-yourself recipes—can help to beautify you from head to toe without costing you an arm and leg.

UN-BEE-LIEVABLE HEALING HINTS TO CATCH

- ✓ While honey is known for common health ailments, it is also helpful for pets, kids, and household uses. . . .
- ✓ Candles, furniture polish, and more are some of versatile virtues of beeswax.
- ✓ Beeswax furniture polish can clean your entire house.
- ✓ Beeswax products, from candles to fun art, can be used by both kids and parents.
- ✓ Gardening tools, golf clubs, and leather goods are all things that can benefit from beeswax, an all-purpose cleaner and preserver of goods.

13

Honey Bee-autiful

If you want to gather honey, don't kick over the beehive.

—Abraham Lincoln[1]

A few years after nesting in San Jose, like a forager bee I found a new home in Boulder Creek in the Santa Cruz Mountains in California. It was an Emily Dickinson–type setting. On the San Lorenzo River, complete with redwoods and oak trees and wildflowers, honey bees and I lived in harmony. A typical Tuesday and Thursday would mean leaving my young furry children—like bee larvae to me—while I traveled to San Francisco State University. Monday, Wednesday, Friday, and weekends were heavenly—a queen bee's existence.

One spring day, after a swim in the river with my two dogs (I had adopted another Labrador retriever), I combined a honey and vegetable oil hair conditioner and massaged the mixture on my long, curly dry locks. Thirty minutes later, I rinsed the goo and shampooed. I dried my hair in the sun. My mane felt soft and silky. I felt like a natural woman again without insect fuzz.

THE BEE-AUTY OF HONEY POWER

I'm hardly alone in discovering beauty benefits of honey and its versatile healing powers from head to toe. As the story goes, Ted Dennard, founder of the Savannah Bee Company, had experienced a beauty brainstorm. One day he was washing his hands at the end of a day working with the hives and noticed how clean and soft they were. He pondered, *How can I bring the beauty secrets of the hive to the market?* After Ted experimented, a line of all-natural beauty products made from honey and other plant and nut extracts came to fruition, thanks to the bees, again. Today, Savannah Bee produces body butter, hand cream and salve, certified organic lip balms, and natural and organic lip tints.

Since honey is a natural preservative and antibacterial agent, it protects and promotes moisture in the skin—which I, too, have experienced. What's more, it's a humectant (an ingredient that holds moisture), something I've used in hair conditioners to help tame my curly mane the same way humidity does in the Deep South and Hawaii.

Eating honey can help you get beautiful on the inside, but treating your body on the outside with the golden nectar can make you look and feel great, too. And honey—from natural stuff in the jar to ready-made honey products—is making a buzz in the present day and has roots from ancient times.

CLEOPATRA'S FAMOUS MILK-AND-HONEY BATHS

Back in the day of Cleopatra, the legendary queen of Egypt savored honey and its beauty powers. The queen allegedly turned to the nectar of the gods for a facial each morning. Milk-and-honey baths were also part of her beauty regime. The idea was that honey was the golden secret to keeping her skin soft as well as defying age.

In the 21st century royal honey beauty treatments have carried over to spas that cater to the rich and famous and include anyone who wants to be treated like royalty for a spa day or week. It's a pampering honey and milk beauty treatment, like the recipe below from Savannah Bee Company, that draws the healing powers to both women and men, thanks to Cleopatra.

Milk-and-Honey Facial Mask

Plastic wrap or warm face cloth
2 tablespoons organic milk
1 tablespoon Savannah Bee Company Wildflower Honey

Take the plastic wrap and cut the corners to make an oval slightly larger than your face. Cut openings for nostrils and mouth. After you make the mask and apply it, you'll be covering your face with the plastic wrap for about 10 minutes.

Add milk to a small bowl. Slowly stir in Savannah Bee Company Wildflower Honey. Mix well and stir until moisture is smooth. It may be slightly runny. Apply the milk mixture to your face with your fingertips.

Set timer for 10 minutes. Put on some soothing music, lie down and cover face with plastic wrap or cloth. When the 10 minutes are up, wipe face with a warm cloth and rinse with cool water. Gently pat skin dry. Finish with your favorite moisturizer.

(*Source:* Courtesy: Savannah Bee Company.)

SPA BEE-AUTIFIYING TREATMENTS

It's no beauty secret that honey combined with other natural ingredients can enhance your blood circulation, zaps stress and anxiety, and makes your skin feel silky. All-natural manuka honey, for one, teamed with other honeys and natural plant extracts and essential oils can help exfoliate, soften, and even make your skin look firmer and glow. And this is why some spas around the nation and world include honey in their spa treatments. Here, take a look at some of the popular ones.

Milk-and-Honey Bath

The treatment begins with a honey scrub, followed by a warm bath filled with milk and honey, and culminates with a light massage. This is a double delight—because it exfoliates and moisturizes the total body.

Manuka Honey Drizzle Body Masque

The spa technician will use bare hands or a spa brush to apply approximately ½ to 1 full cup of product to your skin, from the shoulders down to the feet. It will remain on your skin for about 10 minutes before you rinse it off with a shower.

Orange Blossom and Body Wrap

Enjoy the healing hydrating and conditioning properties of a honey wrap. Treatment begins with an exfoliating full-body dry brushing, includes an invigorating orange blossom and sugarcane sugar foot scrub, and concludes with a yummy application of honey–orange blossom body butter. Fifty minutes.

Manuka Honey Drizzle Pedicure

Savor the pampering of a professional pedicure. Treatment begins with you soaking your feet for 5 to 10 minutes in a basin of warm water and Manuka Honey Drizzle (from Bella Luccè®—www.bella lucce.com).

THE SWEETEST DIY BEAUTY RECIPES

Do-it-yourself products make it possible and easy to enjoy the spa benefits in the comfort of your home. And more people—both men and women—are discovering the beauty benefits of honey, whether it's straight from the hive or comes in a glass jar. Here, take a look at some of the at-home treatments I tried from head to toe and you'll be thanking honey bees forever.

Eyes

Cucumber Honey Eye Nourisher: One of the best things I did one morning was whip up an anti–puffy eye cream with 1 tablespoon aloe vera gel, 2 teaspoons cucumber, peeled with seeds removed, ½ teaspoon chamomile tea, and 1 teaspoon honey. After steeping chamomile tea in boiling water, I set it aside to cool. In my blender, on a low setting, I combined the cucumber, aloe vera gel, and honey, added chamomile tea, and whizzed it till smooth. I put the honey goo under my eyes using my fingers. Ten minutes later, I looked like I wasn't a worker bee.

Skin

Lemon Drop Body Wash: The next morning, I went to the bathroom like a bee goes to a honeycomb and prepared a honey soap of 2 cups unscented castile soap, 2 cups honey, and ½ cup lemon juice—and put it in a plastic bottle and shook it. In the shower, rather than using ready-made honey soap, I used a loofah and washed my body and rinsed. Extra benefit: I got to feel my skin soft and could watch CNN right after without fleeing to a spa.

Feet

Stimulating Camphor and Eucalyptus Honey Foot Soak: That night, I did the favorite thing I did that day: blend 8 cups hot water, 1 cup honey, 2 cups Epsom salt, 2 tablespoons almond oil, and 6 drops eucalyptus oil—and soaked my feet with it. Fifteen minutes later, my feet looked human again.

(*Source:* National Honey Board.)

Both spa treatments and do-it-yourself action work for me. But it doesn't stop there, especially for bold and beautiful people. Prince Charles's wife, Camilla, for one, is noted as having used bee venom—a natural facelift remedy. It's been tagged as "the botox alternative"— combining bee venom, manuka honey and shea butter—and promises to minimize wrinkles.[2]

QUEEN BEE FOR A DAY

A Day in the Life of a Worker Bee

8:00 A.M. Rise and shine. My day starts with getting up and feeding my Brittany duo. Then it's time to make a cup of brewed Italian coffee. I take one cup with a splash of 2 percent low-fat milk (and a homemade honey muffin) back with me and crawl into the warm waterbed. I turn on the tube and log on to the computer to fetch my morning e-mail.

9:30 A.M. Eat a nutritious breakfast. It's time for a light breakfast, such as a bowl of oatmeal or plain yogurt (I no longer eat the kind with high-fructose corn syrup) with fresh fruit and honey on top. (Go to chapter 18: "Ciao, Honey!" for recipe ideas.)

11:00 A.M. Honey shower time. Take a hot shower. First, light a honey-lavender-scented candle. I spray the bathroom with Cuccio Naturalé's Milk & Honey Scentual Spa Elixir. It creates an aromatherapy environment in my cabin-type bathroom. I spray it on a dry towel and in the air. Turn on rock music—something with a beat. This time around I'm using Cuccio's Milk & Honey Sea Salts and want to enjoy the hydrating and exfoliating benefits of milk and honey. I used it on my feet and body. I also use the Milk & Honey Body Wash—it's more fun than a bar of soap. After I dry off, it's a Milk & Honey Butter Blend for my hands, feet, and body. I read that it was "great to use after exfoliating with the Cuccio Naturalé Milk & Honey Sea Salts." It is. I must e-mail a thank you note to Cuccio for taking me back in time to a Cleopatra milk-and-honey experience.

12:50 P.M. Get a move on. It's time for a half-hour swim. In the fall/winter I use the spa resort pool and team it with a hot tub. In the summer, it's a Parks and Recreation pool and the sun is therapeutic. I take 1 teaspoon of raw honey for energy before I go. At home, I use a beeswax hand and nail salve to counteract the dryness from the chlorine in the pool.

1:30 P.M. Eat lunch. I whip up an Italian-style grilled cheese on whole-grain sourdough bread with tomatoes. Afterward, it's time to try a new wildflower honey in a cup of green tea.

2:00 P.M. Walk the dogs. Once back, drink a glass of

spring water (or two) and squeeze fresh lemon in the glass for a tastier beverage.

3:00 P.M. It's time for work. I prefer going to the laptop for articles, desktop for books. Time spent: three hours.

6:00 P.M. It's time to eat. Now that my body and mind have been taxed, it's time to feed my mind, like spa guests who are provided with prepared dinners to die for. Tonight I had a Mediterranean Wrap. (Check out the end of chapter 6 for the recipe.) And that is good for worker bees headed back to work.

7:00 P.M. Have a cup of homemade lemonade. I pair chamomile tea with an exotic teaspoon of honey and ¼ cup of fresh lemon juice and ice cubes.

9:30 P.M. Take it easy. This a good time to de-plug from the computer and phone. I turn on a film and chill. I treat myself to a honey truffle.

11:00 p.m. Prepare for bedtime. I wash my face with honey-oatmeal soap, use honey lotion on my hands. I use a cuticle conditioning butter stick made with milk and honey. I light scented beeswax candles in the bedroom.

12:30 P.M. Sweet dreams. I fix a cup of 2 percent lowfat organic milk with a teaspoon of honey and ½ teaspoon cinnamon. My thoughts are on autumn, when bees produce their honey harvest (and their beekeepers extract the nectar). It's a time when I clean my cabin (piling wood to stocking the pantry) and clean my hive for wintertime, when I bundle up like honey bees and dream about springtime, another season of the honey harvest.

(*Sources:* Cuccio Naturalé and Savannah Bee Company.)

Whatever season or wherever you live, a honey exfoliating mask will rejuvenate your facial skin and you'll feel good both inside and outside. Try this Deep South recipe and enjoy the total queen bee pampering treatment with a cup of tea and honey.

Harvest Pumpkin & Honey Exfoliating Mask

❖ ❖ ❖

1 teaspoon green tea brewed

2 teaspoons pineapple, diced

4 tablespoons pumpkin puree

1 tablespoon Savannah Bee Company Honey

2 teaspoons aloe vera gel

½ teaspoon sunflower oil

4 teaspoons cornmeal

6 drops Frankincense Essential oil (optional)

4 drops cinnamon extract (optional)

Steep green tea in boiling water. Set aside to cool.

In blender or food processor puree pineapple and place in medium-sized mixing bowl. Add pumpkin, Savannah Bee Company Honey and aloe. Mix well. Stir in sunflower oil, green tea and cornmeal. Reserve remaining green tea for another use. Add frankincense and cinnamon. Stir.

Apply small amount of pumpkin mask to cheeks, forehead, chin and neck. Massage in circular motions gently buffing skin. Repeat. Apply more product as needed. Leave a thin layer of pumpkin mask on face and neck for 15–20 minutes.

Rinse with tepid or cool water and pat dry with soft towel. Follow with appropriate moisturizer. Store remaining mask covered in refrigerator for up to 2 weeks.

Makes 4 treatments.

(*Source:* Savannah Bee Company.)

Now that you've got honey beauty secrets, in chapter 14 it's time to bring out the people behind the honey bee, from beekeepers to packers. These folks who love honey are connected to nature—a connectedness like that of a bee colony. I've contacted some unforgettable people who respect sacred honey bees, as well as folks who put it all together so you and I can enjoy honeys in all forms, types, and regions that'll wow you.

UN-BEE-LIEVABLE HEALING HINTS TO CATCH

✓ Honey can help exfoliate, soften, and make your skin and hair look softer.

✓ Honey boasts antibacterial properties, and its ability to hold in moisture can keep your skin, from face to feet, healthy and smoother.

✓ Honey treatments include honey with natural plant extracts, essential oils, and other ingredients.

✓ This golden liquid can help to exfoliate, soften,

and firm skin from head to toe to help both women and men look better, feel great.

✓ Honey masks, wraps, manicures, pedicures, baths, and much more are offered at health spas in America and around the world.

✓ You don't have to go to a spa to enjoy the honey spa beauty treatments, because they can be done in the comfort of your home.

The Busy Bee Workers

*We're all busy little bees, full of stings, making
honey day and night, aren't we, honey?*
—Bette Davis[1]

As a graduate student commuting from my mountain
hideaway to the hustle-bustle of the city, I was on the go,
always working, much like a worker bee. I attended
back-to-back classes from 10:00 a.m. to 9:00 p.m. One
overcast morning arriving on campus I craved a healthy
breakfast. On a shoestring budget I splurged like a queen
bee and treated myself to an off-the-beaten-path bistro
across the street from campus.

The ambiance with lush green plants, incense, and
music in this bistro filled with liberal arts students made
me feel at home—part of a colony. I ordered a bowl of
plain yogurt—not the processed kind with added
sugar—and fresh fruit. The café workers mixed honey
on top of the sweet breakfast treat. I paired this delicious bowl of goodness with a cup of herbal tea and
honey and was in honey heaven. Today I still favor plain

yogurt with pure honey and prefer to eat it amid my own houseplants or outdoors on the deck surrounded by towering pine trees and birds. And I dish out thanks to hardworking honey bees and their human keepers for the goodness of honey.

MEET THE BEES AND THEIR KEEPERS

There are three players in the honey world of human honey producers: hobbyists, part-time beekeepers, and commercial beekeepers. The U.S. Department of Agriculture has estimated that there are between 139,000 and 212,000 beekeepers in the United States.

Hobbyists/Part-Time Beekeepers: The majority, 95 percent, are hobbyists with fewer than 25 hives, and about 4 percent are part-timers who keep from 25 to 299 hives. Together, hobbyists and part-timers account for about 50 percent of bee colonies and about 40 percent of honey produced. The number of U.S. bee colonies producing honey in 2008 was 2.3 million (based on beekeepers who manage five or more colonies).

Commercial Beekeepers: Meet the dedicated keepers with 300 or more colonies. There are about 1,600 commercial beekeeping operations in the United States, which produce about 60 percent of the nation's honey. These folks migrate their colonies during the year to provide pollination services to farmers and to reap rewards of nectar.

(*Source:* National Honey Board.)

THE WORKERS

The top five honey-producing states are North Dakota, South Dakota, Florida, Minnesota, and California—my home state, which makes me feel even more connected to the honey bees and their people. I want to share their unique tales. To me, each of the companies I contacted is exceptional, whether it be for their originality, presentation, reputation, quality, service, or all five traits.

Bee-Pure Honey

Honey History: The Bee-Pure Honey tale is not unusual. Simply put, it was the love of beekeeping in Wisconsin, which began as a hobby, that blossomed into a thriving business.

Healing Powers: The quality products straight from the hive are minimally processed to preserve the real honey flavor. "We add no sugar, water, fructose, or any other junk to our honey," says Thomas Gandia, owner and chief bee wrangler.

My Fave Honeys: I adore a spiced honey in an attractive hex jar. It contains whole spices such as cinnamon and clove. I put it in a cup of hot low-fat organic milk. And in my study sits a file cabinet of some honey treats, such as Bee-Pure honeycomb. As I sit here in my worker bee mode, nibbling on a piece of the U.S. Grade A honeycomb is a strange experience. The sweetness is sublime. I'm getting flashback images of Seth, and I feel like I must look like he did while eating sweets during his morphing phase in the film *The Fly.*

Dutchman's Gold

Honey History: Like Bee-Pure Honey, this company began with bees. As the story is told, Dutchman's Gold began with a swarmed hive back in 1981. Over time the

Van Alten family and company grew to establish 1,500 hives spread on nearby farms in southern Ontario—a province I visited during my honey bee–like traveling adventures.

Healing Powers: Natural honey products are what Dutchman's Gold is all about. We're talking raw, fresh, and unpasteurized honey varietals and honey blends. Also, Dutchman is privy to using beehive products for therapeutic healing and disease prevention. This honey company offers royal jelly, bee propolis, and bee pollen as well as buckwheat honey. From fields of Manitoba buckwheat the bees bring Dutchman Gold—and you—a unique honey. It's dark, rich, and full of antioxidants.

My Fave Honeys: Stocked in my pantry sits Dutchman's products. I love Summer Blossom Honey—it has a mild flavor. It's the wildflower honey that charmed me with its amber color and taste of autumn. The signature cinnamon honey is one honey blend that will be gone before *The Healing Powers of Honey* is completed.

Honey Ridge Farms

Honey History: This is another story about a family business. Located in Brush Prairie, Washington, back in 2004 Honey Ridge Farms was founded. Its mission included providing high-quality specialty gourmet honeys and honey-based specialty foods. "We're part of a long line of beekeepers; in fact, our son is a fifth-generation beekeeper who works alongside his grandfather tending hives," says Leeane Goetz, president.

Healing Powers: It's the quality of Honey Ridge Farm's honeys, being all natural and offering a variety of single–

floral source artisan honeys from the western United States, as well as other all-natural honey-based gourmet foods. The artisan honeys are USA Grade A honey and minimally processed and unfiltered.

Because of their dedication to the apiculture industry and their partnership with local beekeepers, Honey Ridge Farms donates a portion of their profits from their Balsamic Honey Vinegar to help fund research to promote bee colony health.

My Fave Honeys: Honey Ridge Farms' first artisan honey produced was wild blackberry from Washington and Oregon. As a short-time resident of Eugene and Portland and a lover of blackberries, I made this the first honey of the multiple jars I opened. I laced it over a store-bought cheesecake and topped it with sliced almonds. Another favorite food of mine is pumpkin, so their pumpkin blossom honey had me at first sight. I used it baking custard and muffins. It's a keeper.

Laney Honey

Honey History: Moving east to America's Heartland, meet Dave Laney, the founder of Laney Honey, a premium honey company. Back in the seventies, honey was a hobby for Dave, much like other honey entrepreneurs. Twelve years later, his passion turned into a business. Rather than mix in all of their honeys together under one label, they separate their honeys by floral source. That way, Laney Honey is able to offer many varieties of honey. Hives of bees are placed in choice fields of a particular flower in bloom, such as blueberry or clover blossoms.

Healing Powers: Laney honey is unpasteurized, unfiltered, and minimally processed. This is the way to preserve the distinctive flavors, trace minerals, vitamins, and pollen grains found in honey.

My Fave Honeys: Most of their honeys are from the midwestern United States. I did open the jar of orange blossom (from Florida) and used it in a coconut custard pie that I baked. The blueberry is pleasing, sweet, and light. I put a teaspoon on a few scoops of plain Greek yogurt. It was a taste that transcended me from Lake Tahoe to a honey field.

Savannah Bee Company

Honey History: Traveling from the Midwest to the South, I found this unique company, established since 2002. Savannah Bee Company is a thriving company located in Savannah, Georgia. Their mission is to go beyond the call of duty, like a bee colony, to produce the finest, most natural honey products. The Savannah Bee Company has become internationally known for its artisanal varietals, blended raw honeys, and unique body products.

The operation today looks different than when Ted made honey in the kitchen or garage and spent his time lugging hives all over the South in an old pickup. But the passion for bees and commitment to creating the highest-quality products haven't changed a bit. "I just love it," he says. "I can't imagine doing anything else."

These days, the Savannah Bee Company's wide array of extraordinary honey products are sold around the globe, including Australia, Canada, Dubai, and Japan. They also sell their honey products through fine stores such as Dean & Deluca, Whole Foods, Neiman Marcus, Crate and Barrel, and others.

Healing Powers: Ted will tell it like it is. "We spin single varietals out of the comb and into the bottle without blending or processing them." He adds that all of their honeys are hand harvested at the peak of the blooming season to ensure purity, KSA certified, and 100 percent honey.

My Fave Honeys: Here I found a unique company with a gold mine of golden nectar from the honey bee. The gourmet honeys, much like gourmet chocolates, are edgy in presentation, originality, and taste.

Saving the Bees of Tasmania

Enter the world of the Tasmanian Honey Company, which began in 1978, created by Julian Wolfhagen, a native-born Taswegian. Son of a fine wool grazier from the Central Midlands town Ross, Julian grew up close to nature and developed a passion for the environment and the natural world. As a child he would go into the bush with men from the farm to hunt for wild hives and, once autumn arrived, assist them with harvesting the wild honey. He became a beekeeper as a result of saving the bees made homeless by the harvesting operations.

The second, more serious phase of Julian's interest in bees came later. Tasmania was in the grip of a hydro-industrialist mentality, where the loggers of the Tasmanian rain forests were run by the government and wreaked havoc on environmentalism. Julian felt that there had to be a better way for the future of Tasmania and its people and honey bees.

A reacquaintance with bees and honey via a good bottle of mead on a snowy winter's night spent with family and friends in a mountain hut changed the lives of Julian and honey bees. It planted an inspirational seed in the bee man's mind. His idea was to save the bees. And he did just that with the Tasmanian Honey Company, which provides healing honeys around the world.

A CALIFORNIA BEEKEEPER'S BITTERSWEET MEMORIES

Not only did I have the pleasure of speaking with Julian (and tasting his honeys), but another bee guru also moved me with his expertise. Joe Traynor is a former beekeeper who kept around 400 colonies in the 1970s. His words of hard work, like the honey bee workers, produce vivid images of what it's like to be a beekeeper and work hard to pay the rent. . . .

I come back to orange honey occasionally, and it never fails to remind me, not of idyllic hours spent with a gentle breeze wafting through fragrant orange blossoms and the musical hum of millions of happy bees accompanied by a Mozart concerto playing on the truck stereo, but of lifting 100 pound boxes of honey in 100 degree weather in

coveralls soaked with sweat while scores of
angry bees registered their objection to my
intrusion by inflicting numerous stings on
any exposed bit of skin or pinning wet coveralls to flesh, of long nights driving a truck-
load of bees, then sleeping, or trying to
sleep, in the cab of the truck until the bees
could be unloaded at daylight, the angry
buzz of unseen bees echoing in my ears as
they crawled up pant legs and down collars.

OUT IN THE HONEY BEE FIELD
ONE SWEET DAY

I didn't get to visit Tasmania or even go to Bakersfield. I passed on visiting honey shops state by state,
across America, as one individual suggested I do. Nor
did I fly, from bee farm to bee farm, around the world
to meet beekeepers and their honey bees. Still, I did go
out into the field like a forager bee and was treated to a
decadent and soothing honey Jacuzzi bath, and then it
was my day to meet Italian and Russian honey bees face-
to-face. . . .

By 10:00 A.M., both Seth and Simon, my Brittanys, are
dropped off at my vet's kennel for the day while I and
my sibling Bruce set out on our way to Reno for a day of
honey delights. My brother Bruce and I are driving
from South Lake Tahoe. There aren't any beekeepers
around the lake, probably due to the snow. I don't think
the high altitude bothers honey bees.

First stop: Siena Hotel. I recall that in my thirties this
was where I stayed, when it was just a modest but quaint
two-story motel. These days, the Mediterranean-style

hotel is a high-rise, where I stayed next to the Truckee River. More memories are buzzing in my mind as I recall the decadent chocolate bath when I was writing *The Healing Powers of Chocolate*. I sense this will be another sweet experience.

Siena Hotel Spa

One hour later: Spa director Jamie Bell is waiting for us—and we wait in a comfortable relaxation room. Sipping hot herbal tea with Knott's Berry Farm honey while Jamie draws a honey bath is nice. Once again, I am greeted by an oversized bear claw Jacuzzi-style bathtub full of bubbling water (140 jets!).

This time, however, Bella Luccè Manuka Honey is my treat. The lights are dim. The water waits. I enjoy for 20 minutes. Images of Cleopatra came to mind. The Queen of the Nile is claimed to have savored her milk-and-honey baths—and this experience made it clear to me why this is a treat for royalty. This time around it was special but like a sequel, from Chocolate Heaven to Honeyland.

Thirty minutes later: I step out of the tub, get dressed, and am surprised. It's amazing. My skin feels soft. We're talking s-o-f-t. As I wait for my brother to enjoy his honey bath, I am thinking, *I have a new, improved skin—arms, tummy, and legs.* I am awestruck how manuka and orange blossom honeys can affect the skin as much as they do. Next stop to the honey bees is minutes away. . . .

Hidden Valley Honey

Like two disoriented honey bees, we get lost in rural Reno. It is windy. My sinuses are pesky, complete with a headache and sniffles. At last, we arrive at beekeeper Chris Foster's home, away from the feel of the city, and

I feel a calm of country. The atmosphere takes me back to San Jose when I was a kid and fruit trees and prune orchards were still plentiful, not concrete, like in today's fast-paced Silicon Valley.

I am greeted by one nature-friendly man who is a former director of molecular biology at a small firm, where he sat behind a desk looking at DNA sequences on a computer screen. Nowadays, the scientist gone beekeeper and his wife, Karen, are busy living and working with their prized possessions: honey bees. In the house, I am greeted by a German wirehair, a sporting dog that puts me at ease. Everywhere I look there are reminders that I'm visiting a beekeeper. Bee books, fresh fruit, and jars of honey are all over. Chris tells me that his alfalfa from the Nevadan high desert area produces a thick honey that doesn't spoil.

The beekeeper on a mission to expand his 60 colonies to more than 200 explains to me that he usually extracts honey twice a year: "The early honey that is extracted toward the end of June is lighter in color and often tastes distinctly different from the darker fall crop that is harvested before September." He adds that during the extraction process a beekeeper has the option of separating light frames of honey from darker honey and then extracting them separately. Fascinated by the bee-to-honey process, I cannot help but be distracted by the living room window. Outdoors I see a large backyard with bees swarming freely around supers (the white boxes bees live in). A constant movement and buzzing outside in the one-acre backyard has grabbed my attention.

I see bees flying hither and thither. I thought they'd be all tucked away in a hive. Funny, though, the dog isn't bothered by the insects—and neither am I. Chris insists honey bees are gentle creatures. I believe him.

I'm beginning to sense that this day is not going to be a chilling *Killer Bees!* or *Swarmed* sci-fi film sequel. Instead, I'm feeling a sense of calm like Lily Owens, a character who finds solace in the world of beekeeping in the film *The Secret Life of Bees.*

The night before, I watched the movie *Outbreak* (Kevin Spacey's protective gear tears and he's infected with a deadly virus). So, I figure, *Why wear a bee veil? A bee could crawl up my jeans and sting me if it wanted to do it.* I think, *I didn't wear flowery perfume or bright colors like a flower. They'll ignore me.* My brother passes on going outside. (He doesn't like scary movies or honey bees.)

I follow Chris outside. I walk amid the bees. I have entered Beeworld. I secretly wish that I, too, could nurture workers and drones—and queens. That's when he asked me to come face-to-face with his 25 new queens . . . but hey, I think, *I am doing fine. No stings yet. Why push the envelope?* I do not peek inside the containers of buzzing honey bees.

Back inside the house, we chat about local beekeepers, some who rescue swarms and others who sell their bee products as Chris does at the farmer's market. I am given taper candles, lip balm, and a jar of fresh local honey—with promise for helping my sinuses and allergies. Chris tells me that a lot of the honey he sells at the farmer's market is to people who buy the alfalfa honey to stave off symptoms of allergics. I am hopeful that his local honey may give me sinus relief. I want to believe the honey bees that didn't sting me will be my saviors.

Bruce and I pick up the Brittanys, and by six o clock we are back home in South Lake Tahoe. When I walk up to the doorstep I see a big cardboard box with the label "Magnolia Honey." I feel like a bee that is entering her hive. Outside my kitchen window I admire the splash of yellow wildflowers and it makes me think of Italy and wildflower honey. And like a persevering worker bee I found the perfect wildflower honey recipe to take me abroad.

Wildflower Honey-Lace Tiramisu

❖ ❖ ❖

3 cups seasonal berries (reserve ½ cup for garnish at end)

¼ cup of sugar in the raw (brown demerara sugar)

⅔ cup high butterfat whipping cream

¾ cup superfine sugar

3 ounces Italian mascarpone cheese

¾ cup sugar in the raw for mascarpone cheese mixture

2 cups extra strong espresso, cooled

½ cup coffee liquor like Tia Maria

2 Madagascar vanilla beans

½ cup wildflower honey

1 package of ladyfingers or sponge cake

A few sprigs of fresh spearmint

¾ cup sugar in the raw or brown sugar for the berries

In a large bowl stir seasonal berries in the brown demerara sugar. Reserve ½ cup berries for the end. Let the berries mixed with sugar sit at room temperature. Meanwhile, in a mixer whip the whipping cream and ¾ cup of superfine sugar until stiff peaks start to form, taste for sweetness, set aside and keep cool. Take another bowl, combine mascarpone cheese, superfine sugar, 1 cup espresso, ¼ cup coffee liquor and the vanilla beans (scraped well, then chopped). Fold the cheese mixture into seasonal berries. Mix them well but be careful not to break up the berries, using a wooden spoon. Then, fold in the whipped cream to the bowl containing the berries, cheese, espresso and coffee liquor mixture.

Warm the wildflower honey in a double broiler until it reaches a thin consistency. Make layers in the English trifle dish (made of heavy glass) with wet ingredients followed by the dry ingredients; a layer of ladyfinger or sponge cake covering the top of each layer of wet ingredients, honey, then a layer of dry. Repeat. Each layer should look wet. Pour remaining 1 cup of espresso over Trifle bowl with remaining ¼ cup coffee liquor. Drizzle wildflower honey on top. Garnish with spearmint springs. Top with the reserved ½ cup of sugared seasonal fruits. Put in fridge for a few hours to enhance flavors. Serves 6–8.

(*Source:* Warren M. Bobrow, Food Journalist.)

Now that you know how busy the honey bees and their people are, it's time to understand that nothing is 100 percent perfect—not even honey. There is a downside to bees and you should know about it.

UN-BEE-LIEVABLE HEALING HINTS TO CATCH

✓ There are an infinite number of standout honey companies in the United States and around the world; I selected a handful who offered samples and information that taught me more about the health benefits of honey.

✓ Visiting a local beekeeper or going to a farmer's market to purchase local honey is a worthwhile experience . . .

✓ . . . and finding different honeys from different regions can be done via the Internet with the click of your mouse. Go to www.honeylocator.com and enjoy.

Honey Is Not a Buzz for Everyone: The Sting

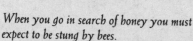

When you go in search of honey you must expect to be stung by bees.
—Joseph Joubert[1]

During my off-school days, one spring afternoon in the mountains, I was sitting outdoors enjoying Mother Nature. A girlfriend and I were surrounded by books, wildflowers, lemonade, and buzzing honey bees. It was a place of sweet comfort to me like when I was a kid. Like happy bees, we were at ease while our two sporting dogs were actively romping around. Her golden retriever and my yellow Labrador were full of energy and quick sprints to catch a ball we'd toss—it appeared like everyone was getting along. Then it happened.

My gal pal's carefree canine dog collapsed. We both shouted, "What happened?" The canine's swollen snout was a sign that a protective honey bee—man's other best friend—was the guilty culprit. One vet visit later: It was confirmed. A bee sting was the diagnosis. Four-leggers and two-leggers can get stung and can have an allergic reaction to bee stings. Most people and pets do survive, as did our dog friend.

The thing is, if provoked, the gentle honey bee—an insect like stinging wasps and biting mosquitoes—can wreak havoc on our furry friends. Once a worker bee uses its stinger in defense its life is over as it once knew it—it expires and goes to bee heaven. A queen bee, however, has a better outcome. She has limitless use of her stinger. So, is the honey bee a friend or foe?

A Pest for Two- and Four-Leggers

Swarming in your home? If the honey bee is setting up house in your house it may seem like you're living with the enemy—not man's best friend. Beekeepers will tell you that the honey bee's instinct is to nest—to live and work in a refuge like I did and do. Honey bees will seek a safe haven, too, such as a hole inside or outside a house or building—often creating a nuisance.

Stinging Pets and People

Although honey bees are gentle, if they are provoked their survival instinct to protect their queen will kick in and they might strike. Some pets can have mild to severe symptoms to a sting, just as a human can. If anaphylaxis (a severe allergic response) occurs, this can be life threatening. Contact your doctor or vet ASAP.

Usually, it takes several exposures before a reaction happens, and it can be mild or severe, like what happened to my friend's canine. There is no diagnostic test for types of reactions, but your veterinarian can make the call during a physical exam. Most dogs allergic to insect stings will develop a swollen face and hives—not the end. Also, the good news is, animals that survive the first few minutes usually return to normal health.

COMMON ALLERGIC REACTIONS TO BEE STINGS IN DOGS

Type of Reaction	Symptoms	Treatment
Mild	Fever, sluggishness, loss of appetite.	Your vet may recommend Benadryl®; and take your dog in for an exam.
Moderate	Urticaria is a moderate vascular reaction of the skin marked by hives, swelling, redness of the lip, around the eyes, and neck. Usually itchy; may progress to anaphylaxis.	A vet visit and exam.
Severe	Anaphylaxis, a, sudden severe	A vet visit ASAP. Your vet will begin

allergic response that produces breathing difficulties, collapse, and other life-threatening symptoms, such as a drop in blood pressure.	ER life support, including administering oxygen and intravenous fluids to increase blood pressure.

There is no way to predict if your pet will have an allergic reaction to a bee sting. If it has happened in the past, make sure your vet knows about it. Since each reaction can become more severe, you should keep epinephrine on hand and know how to use it in case a reaction happens. Ask your vet about an "epi-pen" (a syringe and needle filled with a dose of epinephrine) to keep in your pet's first-aid kit.

(*Source:* Courtesy of PetPlace Veterinarians.)

THUMBS-DOWN ON HONEY FOR INFANTS

From stinging honey bees to infant botulism caused by honey may sound like ideas for an anti-bee sci-film in the works. But in the real world, feeding honey to a human baby is *really* dangerous and should be avoided.

Sweet honey may contain not-so-sweet *Clostridium botulinum* spores. This scientific term means honey can cause infant botulism, because babies less than one year of age do not have the developed gastrointestinal tract of older humans. Honey is safe to eat during pregnancy and lactation. While infants are at risk for infant botulism, adults, including pregnant women, are not.

A Stinging Bee Tale with a Twist

Dr. Tom Potisk, aka the down-to-earth chiropractor, is an advocate of holistic health care. Based in Wisconsin, a bee-friendly state, he recalls an unforgettable past encounter with his sibling and a bee. . . .

I was six years old and it was a hot July day as my sister Julie and I walked hand-in-hand. We were both barefoot after swimming at the neighbors' pool. Taking a short-cut across a white clover covered lawn, hurrying to taste the fresh sandwiches my mom had waiting for us, my youthful contentment was about to be disturbed.

Hearing my sister scream and fall to the ground, I panicked and ran a few steps ahead. Looking back, I saw her swiping frantically at her foot as the culprit, a honey bee, buzzed off. My mother used mud to treat the bee sting.

For years, probably decades after that whenever I heard a buzzing sound my heart would race and my muscles would clench as I looked around in terror. Most times it was a false alarm like a mosquito or harmless fly, embarrassing me if someone noticed my frenzy. As I matured and realized my irrational fear, I controlled it. I enrolled in a beekeeping class. Now I'm chuckling as I write about this and sip coffee with honey from my very own two hives.

GETTING RID OF BEES

Okay, so you get that bees don't like to be provoked and honey is a no-go for babies less than one year of age. But what about honey bees buzzing in your home?

To two-leggers (those who are not beekeepers) honey bees can symbolize flying pests for humans and pets. On the upside, it's time to realize that the *My Girl* film's unforgettable scenario when the character Thomas dies from an allergic reaction to bee stings while looking for Vada's mood ring in the woods is something that happens on the big screen—not so much in real life. It's time to let go of our fear or phobia and face the honey bee—man's best friend.

So, why is it so important to have unwanted bees removed safely rather than just terminate them ourselves? "Honey bees provide a very important service and should not be exterminated unless it is a last resort," says Hidden Valley Honey's beekeeper Chris Foster of Reno. Do not attempt to get rid of bees by yourself. Call a beekeeper to help you safely remove swarms (10,000 to 15,000 bees) or colonies.

Five Eco-Friendly Tips to Prevent Bee Swarms

Local beekeeper Dan Bailey of Sparks, Nevada, dishes out pesticide-free strategies to keep honey bees away from you and your pets.

- Close gaps (i.e., gas line, electrical conduit) on exterior parts of your house.
- Check for improperly installed vents (such as a dryer or hot water heater) on the side of the house, especially on a two-story building.
- Stay on top of maintenance for your chimney. Deterioration (such as failing mortar) provides an opportune home for bees.
- Be aware of outdoor flowers and plants that attract bees.
- Outdoor water dishes for pets are another bee attraction.

CAN BEES CURE ACHES AND PAINS?

While honey bees can cause your home to be held hostage, honey cures are welcomed guests that may move in upon your request. Honey bee guru Joe Traynor recalls that he had resorted to bee venom therapy for his arthritic knee. He received little benefit from the painful therapy. Still, he notes that other people, not excluding beekeepers, believe that bee stings can and do relieve their aches and pains. "The different types of arthritis and the different chemical makeup of individuals could explain why some people react differently than others," he says. It's similar to the fact that there is a wide variation in allergic reactions to stings among both people and pets.

But note, honey bee venom is powerful stuff, which

includes an alleged 40 active substances—including anti-inflammatory substances like melittin and adolapin, which may or may not help lessen pain.[2]

I do not have arthritis but I do know what it's like to have aches and pains after straining a muscle or over-doing it at work or play. When my aches and pains visit me, I do turn to swimming and a hot tub, which can work wonders to relax the muscles and alleviate the hurt. I'll make a note of bee venom and down the line may consider it in my golden years (but hydrotherapy at a royal resort hotel does seem more suited to my queen bee taste).

ROYAL JELLY MAY NOT BE ROYAL FOR ALL HUMANS

From bee venom to royal jelly is quite a leap but still isn't for everyone. While honey larvae and the royal queen bee can dine on royal jelly, it may not be the ulti-mate bee product for you. A small number of people may have allergic reactions to royal jelly. "Asthma and anaphylaxis has been noted in some people after con-suming the honey bee's crème of the crop," according to Ray Sahelian, M.D. He adds that royal jelly has a "blood thinning potential" and so those people taking coumadin (prescribed for a variety of health problems) should consult with their doctor before indulging in the honey bee's "caviar."

Dr. Sahelian adds that bee products—not just royal jelly—may cause an allergic reaction in some people. So, stop use if this happens. If you are pregnant or breast-feeding, consult your health-care professional before using any bee products.[3]

FUNNY HONEY

Tainted honey is no laughing matter. In the news you can find past and present information about foreign firms caught in honey stings. Consumers may be buying honey that is chock-full of chemicals and a mixed bag of contaminants. The bad buzz is, countless honey companies from a variety of countries have been accused of adulterating their honey with cheap additives—not unlike what has happened with chocolate.

Adulterated honey—honey polluted with additives of a foreign or inferior substance, not excluding antibiotics and antibacterial drugs—can cause health problems for people, especially those with chemical sensitivities. Both public health officials and consumers are becoming more aware of this risky business—a honey-laundering game—and measures are in action to put a stop to funny honey landing in your jar.[4]

HONEY AS MEDICINE IS STICKY

Despite the threat of funny honey, there is enough of the good stuff to go around helping you live a long and healthful life. People living at 80, 90, and 100 are proof. Healthy elderly folks around the world dish out credit to the pure stuff, the good golden nectar, for their good health. Still, the school of thought on honey as medicine in the United States is iffy—at best. And the reputation of honey at home in the U.S. as a medicine for pesky ailments and life-threatening diseases doesn't get the attention it deserves.

While anecdotal evidence and stacks of studies in countries around the world show honey has healing powers, medical doctors in the United States, be it the

West Coast, the East Coast, the Midwest or the South are wary about honey as medicine—and aren't quick to prescribe the ancient remedy for heart disease, cancer, or even seasonal allergies.

"Most U.S. doctors are not aware of the benefits of treatment with honey and are not willing to risk the use of this natural substance for legal reasons," explains Dr. Sahelian. He points out that there is the chance a lawsuit could be filed by a patient claiming that the doctor did not use approved antibiotic medications.

"Honey is not available in hospitals and a doctor does not have the option to request the use," adds Dr. Sahelian, who knows that manuka honey has been studied but also knows that honey is rarely used by American doctors. "The role of honey appears to be for the use of diabetic foot ulcers and wound healing," he concludes. And this doesn't surprise me, one who has penned books on subjects from vinegar to earthquake prediction. Nobody wants to rock the world with studies about unconventional theories that don't pan out.[5]

During my visit to Honeyland I discovered that there is a lack of mega-funded studies because pharmaceutical companies haven't jumped on the honey heals bandwagon. *Honey: The Gourmet Medicine*'s author says, "Honey is not a proprietary product—anyone can bottle and sell honey." He believes creating a medicinal honey could be profitable for a drug company.

Meanwhile, people around the globe are using honey as a folk remedy. In 1998, the Australian Therapeutic Goods Administration approved honey as medicine. A company in Australia started marketing medical honey as a wound dressing in pharmacies. Also, in the 21st century European countries sell medicinal honey and some South American countries sell honey for medicinal uses. And in the United States we are moving in the right direction. Manuka is available to us via the Internet.[6]

KEEPING IT REAL AND SWEET

Skeptical doctors aren't going to stop honey lovers, like myself, from using the ancient superfood for its healing powers, especially if it works for them. I do believe that honey is one of the most natural, accessible, and delicious foods in the world, but the fact remains it's not always a miracle worker working solo.

So yes, I do tout keeping it real and sweet can help you to stay healthy—but I do not claim honey can heal every ailment and disease. Incorporating versatile honey into a healthful diet and lifestyle (both inside and outside your body)—in conjunction with conventional medicine if needed—may help you to live a longer, healthier, and sweeter life, just like honey bees being fed a healthy diet and living in a healthy environment.

Healthful recipes, like this real and sweet salad, make a beeline toward good health. But caution: Keep this salad and other food and beverages away from honey bees and their hives for safety's sake of you and yours!

Honey, Mint, and Cucumber Salad

❖ ❖ ❖

Approximately 6
   ounce tub thick
   Greek yogurt
4 tablespoons
   blended clear honey
2 whole cucum-
   bers, chopped

4 tablespoons mint,
   freshly chopped
2 tablespoons lime
   juice
Mint leaves for deco-
   ration

In a large bowl mix together all the ingredients until combined. Transfer to serving
dish, sprinkle with torn mint leaves, and
serve immediately. Serve with thick cut vegetables, such as pepper, celery and carrot,
tortilla chips, or why not try broken pieces
of spicy popadoms for a healthy midday
snack or as a refreshing start to any meal. . . .
Serves 4.

(*Source:* Courtesy The Honey Association.)

If you have a sensitivity to honey internally, it may
work for you topically—for beauty, candles, cleaners,
and other uses. In the future, I sense that honey—the
darker types—will be used more in kitchens and households and medical clinics and hospitals around the
globe. In chapter 16: "And the Bees' Buzz Goes On . . ."
you'll be reminded of how important the honey bee—
our friend, not foe—is to our food chain and maybe
even survival.

UN-BEE-LIEVABLE HEALING HINTS TO CATCH

✓ The honey bee is a gentle insect, but if provoked it can sting both humans and pets.

✓ Do not startle or attract bees if you are in a region where there is a colony or a swarm—more aggressive.

✓ Honey should never be given to infants one year old or younger due to its potential botulism effects.

✓ Bee venom and royal jelly may work for some people and may not work well for others.

✓ Further scientific research is needed in the United States to prove that honey can help heal a variety of health ailments and diseases.

✓ Honey is not a cure-all for every ailment and disease, and hype about its healing powers needs to be brought down to earth. But honey is a gift. . . .

✓ Honey used solo and paired with a nutrient-rich diet can often be a godsend to people in a variety of ways.

And the Bees' Buzz Goes On . . .

The wild bee reels from bough to bough
With his furry coat and his gauzy wing,
Now in a lily-cup, and now
Setting a jacinth bell a-swing,
In his wandering; . . .
        —Oscar Wilde[1]

In my thirties, I relocated to San Carlos on the peninsula in the San Francisco Bay Area. The building I ended up finding comfort and producing articles in for more than a decade was a honey bee's dream hive. It was like a minicolony of artsy, European people living in 14 units of a Spanish-style rustic building. Garden Hacienda boasted Monet-like morning-glory bushes, plum and lemon trees, and a large fishpond full of koi and fresh well water. It was my new home.

But then it happened. The owner of the property was selling the land. Bit by bit, like the fish in Hemingway's *Old Man and the Sea* tale, the gardens were torn apart. The caretaker took a saw to the morning-glory bushes—a honey bees' hangout. The vacant area was to make way for his trailer—a prelude to what was coming next. The back house was demolished and a temporary library took its place. The grounds were being attacked by predators: mankind. Gentrification was happening. A sterile high-rise complex was in the works. And it was time for me, once again, to find a new home, like a bee swarm seeking solace for a safe haven to work.

THE HONEY BEE AND OUR FOOD CHAIN

As I noted in chapter 1, bees make honey and work double shifts as key pollinators for mankind. Did you know that our crops depend on the beekeepers and small honey bee in a big way? Millions of acres of U.S. fruit, vegetable, oilseed, and legume crops depend on insect pollination—and that includes the sacred honey bees. This little insect gives humans gifts from the hive but also helps pollinate our crops, home gardens, and wildlife habitat.

It's been estimated by the USDA that 80 percent of insect crop pollination is done by the hardworking honey bees. If you do the math, that means one-third of the total human diet comes from insect-pollinated plants, including fruits, legumes, and vegetables—all the good, healthful stuff that you and I love and eat each day. And that's not where the honey bees' work stops, either.

The almond crop—prevalent in California—also relies on honey bee pollination. And don't forget most beef and dairy products enjoyed in the United States count on insect-pollinated legumes, such as alfalfa and clover. Fifty percent of all alfalfa seed comes from the Golden State.

"Pollination is not a tangible product of bees, but the rental of bees to pollinate a variety of crops is a major source of income for U.S. beekeepers," says *Honey: The Gourmet Medicine* author Joe Traynor, who runs a pollination (bee rental) and agricultural consulting service in California's San Joaquin Valley. In other words, the value of bees to U.S. crops runs into billions of dollars, much more than the value of the honey produced by the honey bees.

But despite the need for the honey bee—who works a double shift with making honey and pollinating crops—there is a megaglitch that is becoming a growing problem: The honey bee population is declining.

IS THE HONEYMOON OVER?

It's no secret. Beekeepers across America are witnessing the mysterious die-offs of bee colonies. Back in 2006, an apiary owner in Lewisburg, Pennsylvania, made the problem known. Penn State researchers took note of the bee colony numbers' decline, due to a condition now known as Colony Collapse Disorder (CCD). This condition causes honey bee colonies to vanish without a trace—lending to *The Happening* and *I Am Legend* images of thriller sci-fi films of human and animal extinction.

So, what are busy researchers doing during the honey bee crisis? A lot. Penn State University founded a new Center for Pollinator Research, and Penn State experts' concern regarding the threats against pollinator survival led to the first International Conference on Pollinator Biology, Health and Policy, held in the summer of 2010 at Penn State. While the East Coast scientists are busy as bees working out the CCD dilemma, on the West Coast at the University of California, Davis, researchers are also at the drawing board.

UC Davis, just 100 miles south of me in Lake Tahoe, is home to honey bees. Honey Bee Haven is part of pollinator research. It is home to more than 6 million bees, thanks to Häagen-Dazs, which is behind the project. A half-acre honey bee heaven has been created to educate students and the public about our food chain's workhorses.

Bee expert Dr. Eric Mussen gets the importance of the honey bee's contribution to our health, which is through fruits, vegetables, and nuts that are considered health foods. He also knows that people like you and me use honey bee–collected pollens, bee venom, and propolis for their healing powers.

The U.S. Department of Agriculture is also trying to help get a handle on Colony Collapse Disorder. In 2010 it dished out $6 million in emergency assistance to beekeepers who had lost their bees. And scientists are busy at work trying to discover what exactly is causing the vanishing of honey bees.[2]

Theories include climate change, diet, mites, pesticides, and viruses. Also, the stress of traveling for pollination of crops and the usage of cell phones (perhaps due to the radiation) are in the mixed bag of possibilities for why the bees are MIA.

Mussen adds, "None of us know why the bees are not as vital as they used to be. In many cases this may be due to limited access to a good, varied supply of pollens." He hopes in our lifetime scientists will discover what is killing the honey bees. "But," he notes, "even if we find the cause, will we be able to overcome it?"

Bee Culture magazine editor Kim Flottum is also aware that the global plague of CCD still lingers, but he remains positive: "Researchers, beekeepers and concerned citizens all over the world have come together to resolve the health issues our honey bees face."

Adds Flottum: "Researchers have uncovered many of the causes contributing to this problem, and in the process have made significant discoveries regarding honey bee nutrition, safety, genetics and habitat requirements." But the reach-out efforts don't stop there. "Beekeepers, too, have helped by providing more diverse areas to raise and keep their bees, while shielding them from the harsher aspects of modern agriculture, most notably the limited diets monoculture crops provide." In other words, staying clear from the chemical-laden, artificial world of modern agriculture is paying off while hardworking farmers are also trying to help the honey bee crisis in how they protect their crops from the pests and disease with agrichemicals, reducing events where honey bees and deadly pesticides collide.

Save the Honey Bee

What do ice cream and candy have in common? Both sweets have sweet companies that use honey in their products and are behind saving the honey bee. And two rescuers—who produce sweet products using real honey that I've enjoyed like a honey bee splurging on a honey—are supporting the honey bee research at UC Davis.

Häagen-Dazs offers Vanilla Honey Bee ice cream made with real honey and all natural ingredients. They know that the honey bees pollinate one-third of our natural foods, including many of the ingredients they use to craft their 100 percent all-natural ice cream. They are funding research and driving efforts to save these petite pollinators.

Gimbal's Fine Candies in San Francisco (www.gimbals candy.com) is also aware that we need to act to save our hardworking friends. In 2010, they launched a candy dubbed Honey Lovers. These are heart-shaped fruit chews made with real honey and are rich in antioxidant vitamin C. Each serving of Honey Lovers contains 25 percent of your daily vitamin C needs. During the creation of this honey book, I snacked on 16 buzz-worthy flavors topped with honey, including Pomegranate Honey, Honey Dipped Strawberry, Honey Vanilla, and Orchard Pear 'n Honey.

Here are ways we can help keep the honey bee alive and well, straight from Mussen: Devote a portion of your property to growing annual and perennial plants that bloom consecutively over the whole season that honey bees are collecting nectar and pollens for food. Reduce the use of pesticides of all kinds to a minimum. In areas with extended dry periods, supply fresh water in a way so that visiting bees don't become a nuisance. Consider donating funds to bee researchers around the country who are trying to determine the causes of CCD and what can be done to bolster the bee populations.

AWOL HONEY BEES FROM A BEEKEEPER'S PERSPECTIVE

Meet James, a caring beekeeper with 17 colonies, who admits he is not a formally educated guy but is an apt pupil of nature and human nature. He maintains bees and teaches sustainable beekeeping workshops on his 35-acre homestead in the Ozarks, which he likes to call Bee Landing (www.beelanding.com).

He cares about bees and it shows in his words: "My breeder queen is my first love. She is mostly Russian, so she is quite dark, almost black. She is a great queen and very gentle. She has produced nine daughter queens just this year. I whisper sweet nothings in her ear and call her my beauty queen." Here is one devoted backyard beekeeper's-eye-view of the alarming die-off of honey bees. . . .

In my opinion, it is our monoculture society and mentality. We have altered the honey bee and the bee hive to a degree that we have weakened them and made them more susceptible to diseases that they could normally fend off themselves. We have sent them out to gather pollen and nectar in a toxic environment—like orchards with insect disorders that need to be sprayed with pesticides, fungicides, and other cides. How have we altered the bee and hive from what nature intended? Here are my top three concerns:

Super Size Me Disorder: In commercial beekeeping the bees are substantially larger than they are in nature. Larger cell size has allowed mites (another disorder) to run rampant through the hives of the world. Incidentally, you can guess what is used to combat this problem—not common sense or a studying of the bees but a miteicide.

Thinking Inside the Box Disorder: The hive is designed more for the convenience of the beekeeper than for the bees. We have taken them out of their hollow log, rock crevices, and other found habitats and confined them to square, squat boxes. Which means they can no longer build their long and elegant comb, which can be measured in feet, not inches. I'm still trying to learn how confinement affects the bees.

Geographically Challenged Disorder: The bees are mass bred (artificially inseminated) in the southern states and dispersed around the country. This reduces genetic diversity and creates a situation ripe for disaster. Weakened genetics, I feel, are a large part of our current bee crisis.

So . . . What am I doing and what do I recommend you do about it? Stop doing things for the bees! Just stand back and watch nature. Stop all the chemical treatments, and let the bees live or die on their own. The bees that live are your breeding stock, the bees that die are no longer in your gene pool. Go local. If you are not into keeping bees, then get to know and support your local beekeeper, and if you are a beekeeper buy your bees from an existing natural beekeeper as close to you as possible.

UH-OH! CAN CCD HARM THE HONEY YOU EAT?

If Colony Collapse Disorder can wipe out a colony of bees, can it affect the honey you eat? One beekeeper told me the grueling story of how CCD wiped out 50 of his colonies. Naturally, empathy set in, since I've penned articles about dog packs dying one by one to a mystery disease and losing a cat for no known cause. Not to forget the fish I've found belly up in my aquariums for months—and my not knowing the cause of demise. But then, fear hit me. When I opened a jar of a company's honey, I pondered, *Is this honey safe for humans to eat?* Remember, I'm a health author with a vivid imagination and a closet hypochondriac, too.

I contacted bee expert Flottum and posed the unforgettable classic *Marathon Man*'s chilling question: "Is it safe?" This honey bee book author, who keeps 6 to 10 colonies in the backyard, calmed my fear (somewhat) with his words. Flottum does not believe honey itself can be affected by CCD.

"Part of the CCD issue is comb contamination from beekeeper- and farmer-applied pesticides and, though not the sole cause of CCD, is suspected of being a contributor to the stress level in the hive," he says. "To date, honey hasn't been found to have these chemicals involved because the chemicals are soluble in wax, not water (honey), so that's good." And so it seems CCD is a mixed bag of honey bee ailments, not affecting the safety of eating nectar of the gods.

But the glitch is, notes Flottum, the amount of honey produced is affected by CCD because of the die-off in the honey bee population. And if the honey bees don't get help from man, both beekeepers and mankind will feel the pain, because extinction of this key pollinator will affect our food chain and health as we know it.

A NEW CROP OF BEEKEEPERS

Currently, honey bees and beekeepers are being challenged, but that isn't stopping the skyrocketing number of beginning beekeepers from entering the bee culture. Flottum's classes are fuller than they have been in a decade, sales of beekeeping equipment are on the rise, and the sales of bees are not disappearing. If you think the up-and-coming beekeepers are country folk, think again. Meet the new urban beekeepers who live in Denver, New York, and Minneapolis, thanks to the relaxation of laws restricting beekeeping. And many of the people are women. "The greatest drive," says Flottum, "is that people want more control in their lives . . . especially control over where their food comes from."

As the years pass, by 2050 I sense that the honey—not unlike olive groves and cocoa plants and other foods, such as produce—will continue to be challenged by both Mother Nature and mankind. The demand may be higher than the supply, and this could be a good and bad thing. And, of course, I see more of a self-reliance trend happening, where people will make their own honey and grow their own food. It's self-preservation.

Meanwhile, researchers are busy as bees at work to find out why the busy honey bee is MIA, affecting beekeepers' livelihoods, the honey industry, and our crops that are at great risk due to lack of pollination if the honey bee becomes extinct. I do predict that despite today's plight of the honey bee, we will find a way to preserve the insect that is linked to the Earth. And geologist Jim Berkland, a dear friend and octogenarian, penned this poem for me and the sacred honey bee.

To Bee or Not to Bee

A bee in the Bible and its honey fills a need
Fulfilled when willed by beekeepers while
    aging up some mead.
The grape is fine to make some wine but
    honey is the way
To give a buzz so sweetly that you may be
    moved to pray.

The "Honey Wine," historically, dates back
    five thousand years.
When English chose to hit the "sack" they
    didn't pick some bears;
What would succeed was knightly mead,
    fermented and well aged.

But who knew that the New World raised
    no single honey bee;
They came when tourists tired of fighting
    skeeters and the flea;
We bless some bugs, especially when they
    help plants pollinate;
When honey bees arrived, they thrived in
    hives and Utah State.

Acacia or tupelo honey soon found clover
    was the rage;
Then heather or the leatherwood would
    soon complete with sage.
But now the "empty hive syndrome" leaves
    beekeepers little plan;

We hope our honey bees survive, and survive beyond the time of man.

—Jim Berkland, Geologist
Glen Ellen, California

In chapter 17: "The Joy of Cooking with Honey" I am as excited as a virgin queen bee in flight to share cooking tips with you. You may not know that there is a whole new world out there, which you will discover when you realize that yes, you can cook and bake with the golden nectar.

UN-BEE-LIEVABLE HEALING HINTS TO CATCH

✓ There are three groups of beekeepers: hobbyists, part-timers, and commercial beekeepers.
✓ A commercial beekeeper maintains 300 or more bee colonies.
✓ The top five honey-producing states are North Dakota, South Dakota, Florida, Minnesota, and California.
✓ One-third of our diet comes from insect-pollinated plants.
✓ Research is ongoing on the West Coast and East Coast and around the world to find out what is causing the bee colony numbers to decline and how to solve the problem.
✓ A new crop of beekeepers in cities is cropping up as people are taking an interest in growing their own vegetables and producing their own honeys.

The Joy of Cooking with Honey

If you have no honey in your Pot, have some in your Mouth.

—Benjamin Franklin[1]

In the spring of 1999, after two trips to Lake Tahoe, I found a new bee-like refuge amid tall trees and water. On the south shore, an Old Tahoe–style cabin nestled in pine trees caught my eye. Its charm was wood paneling, high beamed ceilings, and a rock fireplace with a quaint kitchen for a queen bee or human with bee-like traits. Once again, and maybe for the last time, I migrated, seeking a home and a place to produce and housekeep like a queen bee.

It was a treacherous trek: about 200 miles in midsummer without air-conditioning traveling through Sacramento (105 degrees). My cat, Alex, 13, and Brittany, Dylan, 9, coped with the challenge of the heat; I lost my 5-year-old beta, Shakespeare, to fish heaven. Still, like a strong and steadfast colony we survived the harsh elements of nature and arrived at our designated destination.

During my past travels and present journey through Honeyland, I've learned that the hardworking little honey bee is a big deal to our health and well-being. Honey is a growing trend in cooking and baking—and people need to get this fact. What's more, honey has the ability to absorb moisture. Simply put, this food of the gods can make your breads, cakes, candies, and cookies keep fresh and moist longer. That's as good as it gets.

MEDITERRANEAN DIET SHOPPING LIST

Did you know that honey can be used in breakfast, appetizers, sauces, vegetables, and entrees as well as desserts? The best part is, by teaming honey with common Mediterranean foods you can enjoy a way of eating for life without dieting. (In chapter 6: "The Mediterranean Sweetener" I provide a chart of specific common foods and flavors of the Mediterranean diet pyramid.)

The first step to Mediterranean cooking is having the right foods right on hand. Below you'll find common staples found in Mediterranean kitchens—straight from the Mediterranean Foods Alliance, an Oldways Program.

On the Shelves

Beans and legumes: chickpeas, cannellini beans, fava beans, kidney beans, lentils, peanuts
Breads: dried bread crumbs, foccacia, lavash, pita
Canned fruit

Canned seafood: anchovies, clams, salmon, sardines, tuna
Canned vegetables
Capers
Dried fruit
Garlic
Grains: bulgur, couscous, cornmeal, farro, millet, oats, polenta, rice, quinoa, semolina
Honey
Nuts: almonds, hazelnuts, pine nuts, pistachios, walnuts
Oils: canola oil, extra-virgin olive oil, hazelnut oil, walnut oil
Olives
Onions
Pastas (all types)
Potatoes
Raisins
Salt: kosher, sea, and iodized
Spices: basil, bay leaves, black pepper, celery seed, cinnamon, cloves, coriander, crushed red pepper, cumin, curry powder, dill, fennel seeds, garlic powder, ginger, oregano, paprika, rosemary, saffron, sage, sesame seeds, thyme, turmeric
Tahini
Tapenades
Tomato Products: canned tomatoes, tomato sauce, tomato paste, sun-dried tomatoes
Vinegars: balsamic, champagne, cider, red wine, sherry, white wine

In the Fridge

Cheeses
Eggs
Fresh fruit

Fresh meat and poultry
Fresh seafood
Fresh vegetables
Fruit juice: grape, orange, pomegranate
Hummus
Lemon juice
Milk
Yogurt

In the Freezer

Frozen fruit
Frozen seafood
Frozen vegetables
Sorbet

HONEY WITH MEDITERRANEAN HEART AND SOUL

Here are some of the best baking and cooking honeys at a glance that you should know about before you fly into your kitchen. (For more information, go back to chapter 7: "Healing Honey Varieties.")

Honey	Flavor	Uses
Alfalfa	Mild	Desserts such as cookies and tarts
Basswood	Fruity	Mixed with butter for a spread
Blackberry	Sweet, fruity	Cobblers, pies, smoothies

Honey	Flavor	Uses
Blueberry	Fruity	Muffins, scones
Buckwheat	Strong	Sauces, molasses cookies, gingerbread
Clove	Sweet	Salads, breads
Clover	Sweet	Glazes for ham
Cranberry	Fruity and tart	Breads, fruitcake, glazes for poultry
Eucalyptus	Strong, earthy	Glazes for poultry, salad dressings
Goldenrod	Floral, spicy	Breads, cakes, cookies
Lavender	Strong, rich	Glazes for poultry, breads, muffins
Lemon	Citrusy, tart	Cakes, cookies, muffins
Orange Blossom	Citrusy, sweet	Glazes for fish, poultry, muffins, pies
Raspberry	Floral, fruity	Cakes, muffins, vinaigrettes
Sage	Herbal	Glazes for meat and poultry

Honey	Flavor	Uses
Sourwood	Sweet, spicy	Breads, cakes, cookies, cream soups, glazes for meat or poultry
Tupelo	Fruity	Biscuits, muffins
Wildflower	Floral, sweet	Breads, cakes, cookies, shortbread

THE HONEY BAKING RULES YOU'LL KNEAD

Finding recipes that use honey was not a task—but it took me a while to get down the tricks of the trade when switching to honey and/or lightening up or losing the sugar for good. You'll discover that foods will stay fresher longer, but also, honey lessens that crumbly texture in cookies and scones. And because of its high fructose content, honey has more sweetening power than sugar, so you'll use less and reap healthier foods.

Here, take a look at five savvy tips, gleaned from Honey Ridge Farms, that'll stick like bee glue once you start cooking with the super sweetener:

1. Substitute honey for up to half the sugar. With trial and error, honey can be switched for all sugar in some recipes.
2. Reduce the amount of liquid in the recipe by ¼ cup for each cup of honey used.
3. Add ¼ to ½ teaspoon baking soda for each cup of honey used.
4. Reduce oven temperature by 25 degrees to prevent over-browning.

5. One 12-ounce jar of honey equals a standard 8-ounce measuring cup.

During my adventures in Honeyland, I got stuck on the Ancient Roman Cheesecake recipe in chapter 2, since it calls for grams in its ingredients. I needed a human converter. Then, I stumbled upon some honey conversion charts that are buzz-worthy.

BEE HONEY

HONEY VOLUME VS. WEIGHT CONVERSIONS

Honey	Cup	Gram	Ounce	Pound	Kilo-gram	Tbl	Tsp
Cup (U.S.)	1	340 g	12 oz	0.75 lb	0.34 kg	16	48
Ounce	0.08	28 g	1 oz	0.06 lb	0.03 kg	1.3	4
Fluid ounce	0.1	42.5 g	1.5 oz	0.09 lb	0.04 kg	2	6
Pound	1.33	453.6 g	15.9 oz	1 lb	0.45 kg	21	64
Kilo-gram	2.94	1,000 g	35.3 oz	2.2 lb	1 kg	47	141
Table-spoon	0.06	21 g	0.75 oz	0.05 lb	0.02 kg	1	3
Tea-spoon	0.02	7.1 g	0.25 oz	0.015 lb	0.007 kg	0.33	1

CONVERT CUP OF HONEY INTO GRAMS, OUNCES, OR TABLESPOONS

HONEY EQUIVALENT MEASUREMENTS

Cups	Grams	Ounces	Tablespoons
⅛ cup of honey	42.5 grams	1.5 ounces	2 tablespoons
¼ cup of honey	85 grams	3 ounces	4 tablespoons
⅓ cup of honey	113.3 grams	4 ounces	5.3 tablespoons
⅜ cup of honey	127.5 grams	4.5 ounces	6 tablespoons
½ cup of honey	170 grams	6 ounces	8 tablespoons
⅝ cup of honey	212.5 grams	7.5 ounces	10 tablespoons
⅔ cup of honey	226.7 grams	8 ounces	10.7 tablespoons
¾ cup of honey	255 grams	9 ounces	12 tablespoons
⅞ cup of honey	297.5 grams	10.5 ounces	14 tablespoons
1 cup of honey	340 grams	12 ounces	16 tablespoons

(*Source:* Courtesy www.traditionaloven.com.)

So, now that I cook and bake dishes with a variety of honey varietals, it's a sweet leap I'd like you to try. Here, this tantalizing recipe from a spa chef will nudge you to join us and enjoy the adventure cooking and baking on the long and winding honey brick road.

Grilled Chicken with Tangerine Honey and Chipotle Glaze, Olive Oil Crushed Potatoes, and Green Beans

❖ ❖ ❖

FOR THE GLAZE
2 cups fresh tangerine juice
5 tablespoons honey
2 tablespoons finely grated tangerine peel or Mandarin orange peel
2 teaspoons minced canned chipotle chilies in adobo sauce (Chipotle chilies are dried, smoked jalapeños canned in a spicy tomato sauce, which is called adobo. They are available at some supermarkets, specialty food stores, and Latin markets.)

Boil juice and honey in heavy, medium-size saucepan until reduced ⅔ cup, about 20 minutes. Mix in grated peel and chipotle chilies.

FOR THE CHICKEN
1 cup fresh tangerine juice or orange juice
⅓ cup chopped fresh parsley
⅓ cup chopped fresh cilantro

1 tablespoon minced garlic
3 tablespoons chopped fresh thyme
2 tablespoons EVOO
2 tablespoons finely grated tangerine peel
or Mandarin orange peel
4 boneless chicken breasts
1 teaspoon coarse kosher salt

Combine the juices, herbs, garlic, oil, and orange peel in a bowl and blend. Add chicken and coat with marinade. Cover; chill at least 4 hours and up to 1 day, turning occasionally as necessary.

Prepare the barbeque grill to medium heat. Remove chicken from marinade; discard marinade. Sprinkle chicken lightly with salt. Grill chicken until cooked through, turning and repositioning occasionally for even cooking, about 15 to 18 minutes. Brush chicken all over with glaze; grill 2 minutes longer on each side.

FOR THE POTATOES

2 cups of fingerling potatoes, washed
Water to cook potatoes
¼ cup EVOO
1 tablespoon kosher salt
Black pepper to taste
2 tablespoons chopped fresh chives

Place the clean potatoes in a 3-quart saucepan; cover with cold water. Place on the stove over medium-high heat. When water boils, reduce to a high simmer. Cook until the potatoes are soft. This should take about 20 minutes. Drain and discard the water.

Place potatoes in a bowl and crush with a fork. Once they are pretty well crushed and chunky, add the EVOO, salt, pepper, and chives. Continue to mix until all combined. Check seasoning as desired.

FOR THE GREEN BEANS
   1 cup green beans such as blue lake
      beans
   Water to cook beans
   2 tablespoons EVOO
   1 tablespoon shallots
   Kosher salt
   Black pepper to taste

Place a 2-quart saucepan on the stove, bring to a boil, and add the cleaned green beans. Cook for 1 to 2 minutes to soften and blanch the beans. Remove the beans from the water and place them in a bowl of ice water to shock them or stop the cooking.

When ready to serve, in a large skillet: Heat the oil, add the shallots and the beans, and sauté over medium-heat, turning often. Once they are hot, add the salt and pepper to taste. Remove from the pan and serve immediately.

TO SERVE

Serve the grilled chicken breast with olive oil, mashed potatoes, and green beans. You may want to coat the chicken with the glaze before serving. Makes 4 servings.

(Source: Jamie West, Executive Chef, Ojai Valley Inn & Spa.)

Now that you've learned everything you want to know about healing honey but were afraid to ask, it's time to bring in the sweet recipes for your sweeter life, in part 8: "Honey Recipes."

UN-BEE-LIEVABLE HEALING HINTS TO CATCH

✓ If you use the right ingredients, the treats you cook and bake with honey will turn out tastier, last longer, and be more healthful than if you used sugar.

✓ Learn the different types of honeys and their uses for different types of dishes.

✓ Do use dark honey for a more healthful recipe and reap the health benefits of its antioxidants teamed with Mediterranean foods.

✓ Discover through trial and error (don't give up, and the changes may be different for you) how to make the switch from sugar to honey in your dishes.

PART 8

HONEY RECIPES

Ciao, Honey!

For the rest, whatever we have got has been by infinite labor, and search, and ranging through every corner of nature; the difference is that instead of dirt and poison, we have rather chosen to fill our hives with honey and wax, thus furnishing mankind with the two noblest of things, which are sweetness and light.

—Jonathan Swift[1]

I recall a few wintertime bee R & R days of house- and dog-sitting for a neighbor at Lake Tahoe. One chilly afternoon, complete with snow flurries, I was relaxing by the warm fireplace, cuddled up on the sofa with my independent Brittany and a clingy rat terrier. I watched back-to-back sci-fi films and sipped tea with honey. I treated myself to the outdoor hot tub and indoor bubble bath while munching on warm homemade scones spread with creamed honey.

That cozy Tahoe setting, complete with sweet treats, brought back memories of my childhood. Companion animals, movies, and special sweet goodies are the good treasures in life that give us those warm and fuzzy feelings on cold days. So during the weekdays or weekends, you can often find me in the kitchen whipping up a new or old recipe—often infused with honey—to feed my body and spirit.

You, like me, have entered your kitchen—a place where you can now savor honey for breakfast, appetizers, main entrees, and desserts. While I sprinkled dozens of tried-and-true recipes throughout *The Healing Powers of Honey*, I saved 50 honey deliciousness dishes (including breakfast, appetizers and breads, entrees and desserts), from seasoned chefs at Canyon Ranch; Golden Door's former chef Michel Stroot, from Belgium; and others.

These good-for-you healing recipes are chock-full of nutritious fruits, vegetables, fish, and poultry. Also, the chefs did not ignore using a variety of vinegars, olive oil, and chocolate. Common Mediterranean foods, including garlic, onions, milk, yogurt, as well as healing spices, are often part of the recipes. For best results, use the honey flavor and brands mentioned in each recipe.

HONEYS AND CUISINES FROM DIFFERENT COUNTRIES

While there are at least 300 honey varietals in the United States, it's believed by honey proponents that there may be 3,000 types around the globe. If you're craving a trip or foods from a faraway foreign country, you can experience exciting tastes and textures without getting on an airplane. Just turn to a honey of the region and pair it with ethnic cuisine.[2]

On the home front in Northern California, the honey people around the globe have spoiled me throughout the research of *The Healing Powers of Honey*. At least twice a week I would find a box of honeys—creamed, honeycomb, jellies, sauces—on my doorstep. My pantry is overflowing with containers of honey—and thanks to one online shop I got to taste exotic honeys not found at my local health-food store, farmer's market, or friendly Safeway. Many of these honeys came from seasoned bee-keepers who had Australian and European roots. And it was a dream come true to be able to taste these delights. Here are two of my favorite honeys from other countries, which are available at www.ChefShop.com:

Italy (Italian Solmielato organic lemon blossom honey). Italy is touted for its pasta, pizza and eggplant parmigiana, and cheesecake. Italian foods can be good for you if you practice portion control—and pair foods with honey such as Italian Solmielato organic lemon blossom honey. Described as "sunshine in a jar," this pure lemon blossom honey will turn rainy days into sunny ones. In the lemon groves on the Tyrrhenian coast of Calabria in May, Filippo Leonardi's bees turn the sweet lemon nectar into a refreshingly zesty yet delicate honey, with a creamy texture. I enjoyed it with my favorite dark chocolate pastry. It also works well with ricotta cheese, an herbal dressing for a salad, premium French vanilla ice cream, and cheesecake.

Tasmania (French lavender honey). Few people know that northwest Tasmania has the largest planting of French lavender in the Southern Hemisphere. French lavender honey is an unforgettable treat. Delicate and fragrant, it is perfect to pair with a scone or French vanilla ice cream. It's an acquired taste—like quality dark chocolate from abroad.

Before You Use Honey

- Honey stored in sealed containers can remain stable for decades and even centuries.
- For practical purposes, a shelf life of two years is often stated. When in doubt, throw it out and purchase a new jar of honey.
- If your honey crystallizes, simply place the honey jar in warm water and stir until the crystals dissolve. Or place the honey in a microwave-safe container with the lid off and microwave, stirring every thirty seconds until the crystals dissolve. Be careful not to boil or scorch the honey.

(*Source:* National Honey Board.)

The Four Seasons Honey Health-Boosting Menu Plan

This four-day honey diet plan is based on the seasons and a nutritious and natural diet plan that uses honey. Yes, like a honey bee, you can have your honey and eat it, too! Recipes can be found in previous chapters or in this chapter. You can mix and match to suit your personal taste.

Winter: Day 1

Breakfast:
1 piece of fresh fruit
1 Cinnamon Honey Bun*
2 scrambled eggs with cheddar cheese
1 glass of fresh grapefruit juice
1 cup of fresh-brewed coffee or tea and honey

Lunch:
2 ounces feta cheese and ½ cup leafy spinach topped
on a whole-wheat pita pocket with ½ sliced
tomato; microwave till crispy and hot
1 cup Greek plain yogurt with slices of fresh
seasonal fruit

Snack:
Nuts
Fruit

Dinner:
Honey-Glazed Game Hen*
½ cup green peas
1 sweet potato

Snack:
A cup of organic milk with 1 teaspoon honey and
cinnamon

*If the asterisked recipes don't include serving sizes, use your
own judgment and stay on portion control watch.

Spring: Day 2

Breakfast:
  2 slices Honey Custard French Toast with sliced
      berries on top*
  Café mocha with skim milk
  1 banana

Lunch:
  Tuna fish sandwich with tomato slices
  1 cup homemade vegetable soup
  1 cup fresh fruit salad

Snack:
  Onion and Honey Bruschetta*
  1 cup fresh lemonade with 1 teaspoon honey

Dinner:
  Honey Roast Lamb with Couscous*
  Tossed green salad with vinegar and olive oil dress-
      ing
  French bread and olive oil

Snack:
  Fresh fruit over vanilla all-natural ice cream or
      cheese drizzled with honey

Summer: Day 3

Breakfast:
Honey Biscotti*
1 bowl of oatmeal and fresh fruit
1 cup coffee or herbal tea with 1 teaspoon honey
1 glass fresh orange juice

Lunch:
Spring Rolls*
½ cup rice
1 cup Greek honey yogurt

Snack:
Fresh fruit

Dinner:
Cobb salad
Mixed vegetables
1 glass red wine

Snack:
1 serving of Strawberry Chocolate Tart*

Fall: Day 4

Breakfast:
Whole-Wheat Cinnamon Apple Pancakes*
1 cup skim or low-fat milk
6 ounces fresh fruit juice
1 cup café mocha

Lunch:
1 slice organic vegetarian pizza with whole-wheat
   crust
1 cup leafy spinach salad with tomatoes, carrots, red
   wine vinegar, and olive oil dressing
1 cup yogurt with 1 teaspoon honey

Snack:
1 cup of cruciferous vegetables, raw
1 cup herbal tea

Dinner:
Honey Mustard Chicken Tenders*
Corn bread spread with honey
½ cup green vegetable

Snack:
1 slice Apple Honey Pie*
1 cup cinnamon tea

A Bee's Buzz on How Much to Eat: Like Europeans, I do not count calories. However, I do rely on portion control—I eat small meals on small plates—to keep my calories in check. (And I do not eat after 7:00 P.M.) Read food labels and you'll see how easy it is to decode one serving size and its ingredients (i.e., cholesterol, fat, sodium, et cetera) and if it's natural or includes artificial stuff. But note, serving sizes also depend on activity level, size, gender, and age. Don't forget, most health organizations recommend five to nine servings of fruits and vegetables per day.

Breakfast

Imagine: You're in a posh Mediterranean-style hotel room. It's quiet. Your eyes feast on the perfect linen white sheets and cozy comforter, with a chocolate mint on your pillow. You smell the fresh, white, fluffy towels and a sparkling clean room—all yours. You're tuned into cable movies, without work to do and with no human or furry children demands. The best part is: room service. In the morning, you know you can reach for the telephone and place your order: French toast with sliced fruit; tea and honey on the side. That was the scenario I experienced— more than once—when I was on the road like a bee used for pollination services during book tours without my high-maintenance Brittanys.

My life in the real world is a bit different. On Sunday morning when I crave that room-service instant gratification thing, I have to put a little effort into getting my breakfast. Sure, I would love to have room service, but DIY breakfast treats like I provide below, such as *Honey Custard French Toast* and *Whole Wheat Cinnamon Apple Pancakes,* have their perks. Note to self: Call our local dog trainer and see how many sessions it would take to train my canine companions to make and serve me breakfast in bed. I'd settle for my sporting pooches to retrieve me a cup of java. Can dogs do that?

Apple Spice Muffins
Bomboloni (Italian Doughnuts)
California Breakfast Bread
Crepes Myrtilles

Honey Biscotti
Honey Custard French Toast
Savannah Bee Breakfast Smoothie
Whole Wheat Cinnamon Apple Pancakes

Apple Spice Muffins

❖ ❖ ❖

Vegetable oil in a spray bottle, or 1 teaspoon vegetable oil
1½ cups old-fashioned rolled oats
1 teaspoon baking soda
2 teaspoons baking powder
1 teaspoon ground cinnamon
¼ teaspoon grated nutmeg
1¼ cups whole-wheat flour
1 cup applesauce
1 Fuji or Gala apple, peeled, cored and diced
4 egg whites, lightly beaten
¾ cup honey
¾ cup raisins
½ cup nonfat plain yogurt

Preheat oven to 375°F. Spray or grease a 12-cup muffin tin with vegetable oil. In a wide-based blender or a food processor fitted with a metal blade, process the rolled oats until they become a fine flour. Sift the baking soda, baking powder, cinnamon and nutmeg into a large mixing bowl. Stir in the whole-wheat flour and oats. Using a spatula, make a depression or "well" in the center of the dry ingredients and add the applesauce, diced apple, beaten egg whites, honey, raisins and yogurt. Stir gently but thoroughly, just until all the flour is incorporated into the batter. Pour the batter into the prepared muffin cups, filling them about ⅔ full.

Bake for 25 minutes, or until the tops of the muffins

are lightly browned and a toothpick inserted into the center of a muffin comes out clean. Turn onto a wire rack; serve warm or let cool. Makes 12 muffins.

(*Source:* Reprinted with permission from *The Golden Door Spa Cooks Light & Easy* by Chef Michel Stroot, published by Gibbs Smith, 2003.)

Bomboloni (Italian Doughnuts)

❖ ❖ ❖

1/2 cup milk, lukewarm
1 package dry yeast
2 1/2 cups flour
1/2 teaspoon salt
1/4 cup sugar

1 teaspoon vanilla
2 eggs (or 4 egg whites)
1/4 cup Marsala Olive Oil
Olive oil for cooking
1/2 to 1 cup honey for drizzling

In small mixing bowl add milk; sprinkle with yeast. Let stand about 5 minutes until dissolved. In another mixing bowl, combine flour, salt and sugar, make well in center. Pour in yeast mixture, vanilla, eggs and olive oil. Stir until dough holds together.

On lightly floured board, knead dough until smooth and elastic. Place back in bowl, cover and let rise in a warm place until doubled. Turn dough out on lightly floured board, cut dough into walnut size pieces, and shape into balls. Flatten slightly, cover, let stand 10 minutes. In small saucepan, add 2 inches olive oil, heat to 350°F. Cook dough pieces until golden brown on all sides. Remove with slotted spoon. Place on clean paper towel lined baking sheet. Arrange on serving plate.

Bombolini may be filled with a small amount of custard or jam. Sprinkle with cinnamon. Drizzle with honey. [Good choices are wildflower and clover varietals.] Dough may be cut with doughnut cookie cutter. Serves 40 to 50.

(*Source:* Courtesy Gemma Sanita Sciabica, *Baking with California Olive Oil: Dolci and Biscotti Recipes.*)

California Breakfast Bread

❖ ❖ ❖

½ cup Sue Bee Honey®
2 cups low-fat buttermilk
¼ cup raisins
1 cup all-purpose flour
½ cup wheat germ

1½ cups whole wheat flour
1 teaspoon salt
2 teaspoons baking soda
¼ cup molasses
¼ cup chopped nuts

Preheat oven to 400°F. Prepare nonstick loaf pan by spraying with cooking spray. Mix together all ingredients and pour into prepared pan. Place pan in oven and lower oven temperature to 350°F. Bake for 1 hour. Turn loaf out on rack and cool. Allow bread to cool at least 8 hours before slicing and toasting this bread.

(*Source:* Courtesy: Sue Bee Honey®)

Crepes Myrtilles

❖ ❖ ❖

FOR THE PANCAKES

2 ounces flour
Pinch of salt
1 egg, beaten

¼ pint milk
1 ounce butter

FOR THE FILLING

2 ounces butter
2 ounces caster sugar
4 teaspoons clover honey

7 ounces blueberries
Splash of cassis or cognac

First make the pancakes. Place flour and salt in a bowl and beat in egg. Gradually add milk and beat more to give a smooth, thin batter—it should be the consistency of single cream. Melt a little butter in a pan and add a scant ladleful of batter. Swirl around to coat the bottom of the pan thinly. Cook over medium heat until the underside is beginning to brown. Flip over and cook other side. Repeat with remaining butter and batter. Cool pancakes.

Fold pancakes in half, then in half again to give a triangular pocket. Heat 1 ounce butter in a pancake pan and add 1 ounce sugar. Bubble to dissolve sugar and make a syrup. Spoon buttery mix over and heat through. Add half honey and just melt—do this at the last minute as honey can scorch. Repeat with remaining ingredients, pancakes and blueberries. Serve immediately finished with a splash of cassis or cognac. Serves 4.

(*Courtesy:* The Honey Association.)

Honey Biscotti

❖ ❖ ❖

1/2 cup sugar
3 1/2 cups flour
2 teaspoons baking powder
1 teaspoon salt
2 teaspoons cinnamon
1/2 teaspoon cloves
1 1/4 teaspoons nutmeg
3 eggs (or 6 egg whites)
1/3 cup Marsala Olive Oil
1 cup honey
1/2 teaspoon almond extract
1/2 cup almonds sliced or
　chopped
3/4 cup macadamia or walnuts
　chopped
1/2 cup hazelnuts chopped
　coarsely
1/2 cup maraschino cherries
　chopped small
2 tablespoons maraschino
　cherry syrup if needed
4 ounces semisweet baking
　chocolate melted, cooled
Grated peel of 1 or 2 oranges

Sift dry ingredients, including orange peel [except cherries and hazelnuts], into a mixing bowl. Make well in center. In another bowl add eggs, oil, honey and almond extract; stir. Pour egg mixture into dry ingredients. Stir until dough holds together. Add nuts and cherries/syrup. Place dough on floured board, knead, and cut into 6 pieces. Roll each piece into a 2-by-12-inch log. Place logs on foil lined greased baking sheet, 4 inches apart. Bake in a 350°F oven for about 20 minutes or until firm to the touch. Remove from oven and cool about 15 minutes. With serrated knife cut logs diagonally into 1/2 inch thick slices with a gentle sawing motion. Place biscotti back on baking sheet, cut side down. Bake 8 to 10 minutes to crisp. Makes 70–80.

(*Source:* Courtesy Gemma Sanita Sciabica, *Baking with California Olive Oil: Dolci and Biscotti Recipes.*)

Honey Custard French Toast

❖ ❖ ❖

½ cup honey
1 cup milk
6 eggs
1½ teaspoons cinnamon

⅛ teaspoon salt
12 slices (¾-inch thick) French
    bread
Butter
Honey and toasted pecan pieces

In large bowl, beat together honey, milk, eggs, cinnamon and salt. Dip bread slices in egg mixture, turning to coat. Brown soaked slices in butter over medium heat, turning once. Serve with honey and sprinkle with pecans, if desired.

(*Source:* National Honey Board.)

Savannah Bee Breakfast Smoothie

❖ ❖ ❖

2 cups milk
¼ cup Savannah Bee
    Company Orange Blossom
    Honey
1 banana

½ cup orange juice
¼ cup powdered milk
¼ cup wheat germ
Ice

Combine ingredients in a blender and mix well.

(*Source:* Courtesy Savannah Bee Company.)

Whole Wheat Cinnamon Apple Pancakes

❖ ❖ ❖

2 cups whole wheat flour
4 teaspoons baking powder
1 teaspoon ground cinnamon
½ teaspoon salt
2 tablespoons Sue Bee Honey®

2 eggs
2 cups skim milk
1 tablespoon olive oil
1 medium apple, chopped

Combine first four ingredients in large bowl.

Combine next four ingredients in separate bowl, and stir into dry ingredients just until moistened.

Stir in chopped apple.

Pour batter by ⅓ cupfuls onto a hot nonstick skillet coated with nonstick cooking spray; turn when bubbles form on top and cook until second side is golden brown.

(*Source:* Courtesy Sue Bee Honey®)

Appetizers and Breads

More than 20 years ago, my life was unstable. My new landlord didn't allow pets, so I decided to give up my four-year-old gray and white cat, Gandalf. I found a good home for him 75 miles away. Two days after I dropped him off, it hit me like a bolt of lightning. I had made a huge mistake! I traveled back to Gandalf's home and brought a gift of freshly baked banana nut bread (made with honey) and begged his "new" owners to let me have my precious cat back. One hundred and fifty miles and another house move later, I knew in my heart I made the right decision. Gandalf the wizard-like cat became my Rock of Gibraltar for 18 years.

The secret to incorporating the gift of appetizers and breads into your life is to include honey. For instance, drizzling honey on a piece of *Onion and Honey Bruschetta* or spreading rare white honey on a slice of warm, fresh tropical *Banana Nut Bread* would make a beekeeper or bees smile.

Apricot Honey Bread
Banana Nut Bread
Cinnamon–Chocolate Chip Scones
Dates and Honey Bread
Fig Bread
Italian Croissants with Honey Pecan Filling
Onion and Honey Bruschetta

Apricot Honey Bread

❖ ❖ ❖

3 cups whole wheat flour
3 teaspoons baking powder
1 teaspoon ground cinnamon
½ teaspoon salt
¼ teaspoon ground nutmeg
1¼ cups 2 percent low-fat
1 cup honey

1 egg, slightly beaten
2 tablespoons vegetable oil
1 cup chopped dried apricots
½ cup sunflower seeds,
   chopped walnuts, or
   chopped almonds
½ cup raisin

Combine dry ingredients [except for apricots, sunflower seeds, and raisins] in large bowl. Combine milk, honey, egg, and oil in separate large bowl. Pour milk mixture over dry ingredients and stir until just moistened. Gently fold in apricots, sunflower seeds, and raisins. Pour into greased 9-by-5-by-13–inch loaf pan. Bake at 350°F for 55 to 60 minutes or until wooden pick inserted in the center comes out clean. Makes 12 servings.

(*Source:* National Honey Board.)

Banana Nut Bread

❖ ❖ ❖

⅓ cup sugar
½ cup butter
2 eggs
⅓ cup honey
3 tablespoons milk
1 teaspoon vanilla

½–1 cup nuts
2 cups flour
¼ teaspoon salt
4 crushed bananas
1 teaspoon baking soda

Cream sugar and butter, add eggs, and beat. Combine rest of ingredients. Pour into well-greased loaf pans. Bake 45–50 minutes in 350°F oven. After baking, let cool for 5 minutes and remove from pans. Makes 2 regular-sized loafs.

(*Source:* Courtesy Honey Ridge Farms.)

Cinnamon–Chocolate Chip Scones

❖ ❖ ❖

2½ cups whole-wheat flour
¼ cup white sugar
1 teaspoon baking powder
½ teaspoon baking soda
1½ teaspoons cinnamon
¼ cup European-style butter (cold cubes)
¾ cup 2 percent low-fat buttermilk

¾ cup low-fat plain yogurt
1 brown egg
¼ cup clover honey
1 cup 70 percent cocoa content chocolate chips or premium baking semi-sweet chocolate chips
Organic raw sugar
¾ cup almonds, sliced

Preheat oven to 400°F. In a bowl, mix flour, sugar, baking powder and soda, and cinnamon. Add chunks of butter, sliced in small squares. In another bowl, combine buttermilk, yogurt, egg, and honey and stir. Combine wet ingredients with dry. Stir until a dough-like mixture forms. Fold in chips. Drop large spoonfuls of dough onto parchment-lined cookie sheet. Sprinkle with raw sugar. Bake for 12–15 minutes. Cool. Slice in half and spread with creamed honey or cream cheese. Serves 12 medium scones.

Dates and Honey Bread

❖ ❖ ❖

2½ cups all-purpose flour
2 teaspoons baking powder
1 teaspoon baking soda
¾ teaspoon salt
1 teaspoon ground cinnamon
¼ teaspoon ground allspice
1 teaspoon ground nutmeg
¼ teaspoon ground ginger

¾ cup pitted and chopped
    dates or raisins
½ cup pecans, chopped
¾ cup buttermilk
¾ cup honey
¼ cup vegetable oil
2 tablespoons molasses
1 egg

In large mixing bowl, blend flour, baking powder, baking soda, salt and spices. Stir in dates or raisins and nuts; set aside. Beat together buttermilk, honey, oil, molasses and egg. Add liquid ingredients to dry ingredients, stir until just mixed. Spray a 9-by-5-inch loaf pan with nonstick cooking spray. Pour in batter. Bake at 325°F for 55 to 60 minutes or until toothpick inserted in center comes out clean. Cool for 20 minutes. Remove from pan and cool on wire rack. Makes 1 loaf.

(*Source:* National Honey Board.)

Fig Bread

❖ ❖ ❖

½ cup water, lukewarm
½ cup orange juice, room
    temperature
1 package dry yeast
2½ cups flour

¼ teaspoon fiori di Sicilia (or
    1 teaspoon orange extract)
1 egg white
½ teaspoon salt (or to taste)
¾ cup dried figs, chopped

1 teaspoon sugar
3 tablespoons Marsala Olive
 Oil
4 tablespoons honey

½ cup pine nuts (or nuts of
 your choice, chopped)
Grated peel of one orange

In a mixing bowl add water, orange juice, yeast, ½ cup flour and sugar, stir. Let stand about 15 minutes. Stir in remaining flour, olive oil, honey, fiori di Sicilia, egg white and salt. Turn onto floured board, knead until smooth. Return to bowl, cover, and let rise in a warm place until doubled. Place dough on floured board, pat down, cover with figs, pine nuts and grated orange peel. Work figs into dough. At this point the dough may be made into a round loaf or into a braid. Place on oiled baking pan. Let rise covered, until doubled. Drizzle top with oil. May be baked in the pan or on a baking stone placed in oven. Slide risen dough onto stone. Bake in 375°F oven for 25 to 35 minutes or until golden brown. Cover with foil loosely if browning too quickly. Remove from oven and cool on wire rack. Serve with meals or for a snack. Top slices with a drizzle of olive oil or spread with ricotta and honey. Makes one loaf.

VARIATION

Substitute pitted prunes, raisins, dried pineapple chopped, or dried fruit of your choice for figs. Note: For braid, cut dough into 3 even pieces. Roll each piece to about 14 inches long. Place rolls side by side on greased baking sheet. Braid rolls, pinch each end together; tuck under braid. To form a wreath, bring ends together and seal both ends.

(*Source:* Courtesy Gemma Sanita Sciabica, *Cooking with California Olive Oil: Treasured Family Recipes.*)

Italian Croissants with Honey Pecan Filling

❖ ❖ ❖

DOUGH

1 package dry yeast
1½ cups milk, lukewarm
2 ½ to 3 cups flour
1 teaspoon salt

1 egg white
⅓ cup cornstarch
4 tablespoons Marsala Olive Oil

HONEY PECAN FILLING

¼ cup honey
1 cup pecans, finely chopped

½ teaspoon cinnamon
½ cup currants

In large mixing bowl, dissolve yeast in milk. Stir in flour, salt, egg white, cornstarch and olive oil until dough holds together. On floured surface, knead dough until smooth. Cover and let rise in a warm place until doubled, about 1 hour. On lightly floured surface pat dough down to about a 12-inch round. Cut into 12 pie-shaped pieces. Place about 1 tablespoon filling on wide end of each piece. Starting from wide end, roll into a crescent placing point underneath. Place on greased baking sheets, brush with egg white, and sprinkle with seeds. Let rest covered about 20 minutes. Bake in a 375°F oven for 20 minutes or until golden brown. Makes 12.

(*Source:* Courtesy: Gemma Sanita Sciabica, *Cooking with California Olive Oil: Popular Recipes.*)

Onion and Honey Bruschetta

❖ ❖ ❖

¼ cup Sciabica's or Marsala
   Extra Virgin Olive Oil
1 onion, sliced thin
6 slices (½ inch thick)
   ciabatta bread
1 cup pesto

6 tablespoons honey
6 slices turkey, lean, low salt
6 slices Camembert or Gruyère
   cheese
6 slices beefsteak tomatoes

In medium skillet add olive oil and onion; cook until golden. Remove from heat; cool. Grill or toast bread until golden. Spread with pesto; drizzle with honey on each slice. Add onion evenly between slices, top with turkey and cheese slices. Place tomatoes over cheese; drizzle with olive oil. Yum! Makes 6.

(*Source:* Courtesy Gemma Sanita Sciabica, *Cooking with California Olive Oil: Recipes from the Heart for the Heart.*)

Salads

As a teenager I entered Vegetarianland. One Thanksgiving I protested and resisted tasting the big bird. I said, "I don't eat anything with eyes." My mother was shocked. I didn't mean to hurt her feelings, but I was on a mission to eat vegetables, fruits, breads, and anything but meat or poultry. One evening in the kitchen the rest of my family enjoyed a Swiss steak dinner while I munched on a tossed green salad and potatoes. That is a feast that I still enjoy to this day. I'm not talking about a salad with iceberg lettuce and sliced tomatoes. It's serious salad time, with a variety of veggies, dark leafy greens, nuts, and a vinegar and olive oil dressing. This was a no-nonsense salad to live for—a pile of greens that any rabbit would be pleased to see. Sure, it was a rebellion in the suburbs where families ate meat and potatoes, but for me it was the road that led to my Mediterranean diet and lifestyle.

In France and Italy, salads are enjoyed for lunch and before dinner or as a main entree dish. Not only are salads healthy and they contain less fat and calories (especially if you don't drown them in a high-fat dressing), but they can fill you up, too. Also, adding fresh seasonal vegetables and herbs kicks up the taste more than a notch. *Grilled Vegetable Salad* and *Arugula Salad with Honey-Herb Dressing* are two recipes in this section that'll get you rethinking the power of salads.

*Almond-Crusted Shrimp Salad with
Citrus Dressing
Apple and Toasted Pecan Salad with
Honey Poppy Seed Dressing
Arugula Salad with Honey-Herb Dressing
Bang Bang Chicken Salad
Grilled Vegetable Salad
Lentil Salad
Roasted Salmon Salad with
Honey Mustard Vinaigrette*

Almond-Crusted Shrimp Salad with Citrus Dressing

❖ ❖ ❖

*Juice of 2 limes, divided
2 tablespoons soy sauce
2 cloves garlic, smashed
1 pound medium raw shrimp,
de-veined, tails-on
½ cup raw almonds
3 tablespoons flour
¼ teaspoon salt
2 egg whites, lightly beaten*

*4 tablespoons Delicate Extra
Virgin Olive Oil, such as
Arbequina
2 tablespoons Clementine
Olive Oil
2 teaspoons honey
8 cups mixed greens
2 cups cherry tomatoes,
halved
1 ripe avocado, diced*

Combine half of the lime juice, soy sauce and garlic in a bowl. Add shrimp and toss with hands to coat well.

Set aside. Using a blender or food processor, crush almonds (in the absence of a blender or food processor, this can be done by placing the almonds in a plastic bag and crushing with a mallet or rolling pin). Combine almonds in a bowl with flour and salt. Set aside. Set up an assembly line of seasoned shrimp, the egg whites, and the almond-flour mixture. Dip each shrimp in the egg white and then dredge in the almond-flour mixture. Set on clean plate. Heat the Extra Virgin Olive Oil in a large frying pan over medium-high heat. Cook shrimp for 2–3 minutes on each side, or until the outside of the shrimp becomes brown and crisp. Drain on paper towels. Whisk together the remaining lime juice, Clementine Olive Oil and the honey. Drizzle over mixed greens, tomatoes and avocado. Toss well. Arrange the dressed salad on plates. Top each salad with the warm shrimp and hot sauce or red chili flakes if desired. Serves 4.

(*Source:* Courtesy The Olive Press.)

Apple and Toasted Pecan Salad with Honey Poppy Seed Dressing

❖ ❖ ❖

½ cup Sue Bee Honey®
2 tablespoons poppy seeds
½ cup cider vinegar
1 Fuji apple
1 6-ounce package feta cheese
¼ teaspoon pepper

1 head romaine lettuce
¾ cup vegetable oil
1 cup pecans
½ cup dried cranberries
1 small red onion

Proportion salad ingredients to personal taste. Combine dressing ingredients and mix thoroughly. Toss dressing with salad just before serving. Serves 6.

(*Source:* Courtesy Sue Bee Honey®)

Arugula Salad with Honey-Herb Dressing

❖ ❖ ❖

4 cups arugula leaves
1 cup cherry tomatoes
1 cup mushrooms, sliced
1 cup Parmesan cheese, sliced
   Croutons, or toasted bread
   slices

¼ cup lemon juice
2 tablespoons honey
2 tablespoons olive oil
½ teaspoon dried basil
½ teaspoon dried coriander
Salt to taste

In a large bowl, combine salad ingredients, cover, and refrigerate. Combine all the ingredients of the dressing in a jar, close jar, and shake until well blended. Sprinkle with Parmesan, pour dressing over, and toss lightly.

(*Source:* National Honey Board.)

Bang Bang Chicken Salad

❖ ❖ ❖

FOR THE DRESSING
3 tablespoons soy sauce
Juice of 2 limes
2 tablespoons freshly grated
   root ginger

2 green chilies, finely chopped
3 tablespoons clear honey
4 tablespoons nut oil

FOR THE SALAD
1 cucumber
1–2 large carrots
4 spring onions, finely
   chopped
Chinese leaf cabbage, shredded

2 tablespoons sesame oil
1 clove garlic, crushed
Pinch of dried chili flakes
2 boneless skinless chicken
   breasts, sliced

Place the dressing ingredients in a screw-topped jar and shake well to mix together. To prepare salad, slice the cucumber, carrots and spring onions into fine matchsticks, mix with shredded Chinese leaf cabbage, and transfer to a serving plate or bowl. Heat the oil and add the garlic, chili flakes, and sliced chicken. Stir-fry until browned and cooked through. Add to the salad and toss through the prepared dressing. Serve immediately. Serves four.

(*Source:* Courtesy The Honey Association.)

Grilled Vegetable Salad

❖ ❖ ❖

2 tablespoons clear honey
2 tablespoons balsamic
  vinegar
3 tablespoons olive oil
2 tablespoons torn basil leaves
  (optional)
4 ounces Mozzarella cheese,
  cubed
1 pound plum tomatoes,
  chopped

2 small aubergines
  (eggplants)
Rock salt and black pepper
Olive oil for drizzling
1 red pepper
1 yellow pepper
8 ounces baby or small
  courgettes [zucchini]

Mix together the dressing ingredients in a large bowl and add Mozzarella and tomatoes. Leave to marinate. Meanwhile, thinly slice aubergines, place on baking sheet, season, and drizzle with olive oil. Place under a preheated grill until crisp. Repeat, cut the peppers into chunks, and slice the courgettes lengthways. Add grilled vegetables to Mozzarella and tomatoes and serve immediately. Serves 4–6.

(*Source:* Courtesy The Honey Association.)

Lentil Salad

❖ ❖ ❖

2 cups lentils, cooked
2 tomatoes, chopped
2 cups broccoli flowerets,
   cooked crisp tender
1 cup orzo pasta, cooked, cooled
2 green onions (white part)
   sliced thin
½ cup raisins or dates, chopped
1 teaspoon fresh ginger, grated

2 garlic cloves, minced
1½ cups chicken, turkey,
   cooked, cubed
1 cup fresh mushrooms,
   cooked, quartered
1 cup carrots, shredded
1 cup peas, green beans or
   corn, cooked crisp tender
1 cup feta cheese, crumbled

DRESSING

⅓ cup Marsala Olive Fruit
   Oil
⅓ cup orange juice
¼ cup lime or lemon juice
2 tablespoons fresh tarragon or
   cilantro, chopped

1 cup fresh basil or mint,
   chopped
¼ cup honey
1 tablespoon peanut butter

Combine dressing ingredients and blend. Add all salad ingredients in large, shallow serving bowl. Pour on dressing and toss gently. Serves 4–6.

(*Source:* Courtesy Gemma Sanita Sciabica, *Cooking with California Olive Oil: Treasured Family Recipes.*)

Roasted Salmon Salad with Honey Mustard Vinaigrette

❖ ❖ ❖

DRESSING

½ cup balsamic vinegar
2 tablespoons dried cranberries
8 dried apricots, thinly sliced

2 teaspoons Dijon mustard
2 teaspoons honey
1 tablespoon extra virgin olive oil

SALAD

1 pound salmon fillet, cut into 4 equal portions
½ teaspoon sea salt
¼ teaspoon freshly ground black pepper
8 cups spinach, washed

2 cups thinly sliced yellow squash
2 cups thinly sliced red bell pepper
3 tablespoons toasted chopped pecans

Preheat oven to 425°F. Lightly coat a sheet pan with canola oil.

In a small saucepan, combine balsamic vinegar, cranberries, and apricots. Bring to a boil and simmer for 5 minutes. Strain and reserve liquid and fruit.

Season salmon fillets with salt and pepper. Place on sheet pan and bake for 5 minutes or until just cooked through.

Place 2 cups spinach on each plate. Top with ½ cup each squash and bell pepper. Place salmon fillet on each salad and sprinkle with 2 teaspoons pecans. Top with 2 tablespoons dressing and 1 tablespoon of reserved fruit. Serves 4.

(*Source:* Canyon Ranch.)

Entrees

Years ago, I had my heart set on a picture-perfect honey-roasted turkey. I purchased a pricey bird—a big one. Once home, I eagerly washed it. I groomed it for baking. Then, without reading instructions or having the pro chef's know-how, I simply spread clover honey without any other ingredients on top of the poultry. I was in love with an after picture in my mind: a roasted turkey with stuffing and vegetables on a platter. I didn't have a clue about how honey would affect an uncooked 16-pound bird and assumed the before picture was good to go into the oven.

Within a half hour, I smelled smoke. When I ran into the kitchen it was smoke filled. Accidentally I had turned the oven on to Broil. I was afraid to open the oven door to see the damage. I had a burned bird on my hands. In between tears and feeling like I lost my best friend, I began damage control. *I can salvage my turkey and try again—without a honey glaze,* I thought. The end result: My turkey platter was doable, but it wasn't the picturesque dinner of my dreams. I blamed my mistake on the honey and my ignorance of how to use it.

Today, I know that honey cooks faster than other basting ingredients and if you use this all-natural sweetener it's a good thing to combine it with other ingredients, too, for more flavor. There are recipes such as *Asian Honey-Tea Grilled Prawns* and *Honey Roast Lamb with Couscous* that show how to prepare and bake meat with special honeys that have given me a new lease on baking entree masterpieces from start to finish—without having to call the fire department or dry any tears.

Acacia Duck
Asian Honey-Tea Grilled Prawns
Buckwheat Honey Roasted Chicken Breasts with
Black Truffle Oil, Yukon
Gold Hash, and Grilled Asparagus
Grilled Honey-Glazed Pork Tenderloin with Onions
Honey-Glazed Game Hen
Honey Mustard Chicken Tenders
Honey Roast Lamb with Couscous
Marinated Mackerel
Pomegranate Glazed Chicken
Spicy Honey-Pepper Glazed Snapper
Spring Rolls

Acacia Duck

❖ ❖ ❖

4 medium duck breasts,
   trimmed
4 tablespoons sunflower oil
1 tablespoon Chinese Five Spice
1 tablespoon Acacia honey
2-inch piece of ginger, peeled
   and in matchsticks

2 fat cloves garlic, trimmed
   and sliced in strips
2 spring onions, trimmed and
   sliced in strips
8 ounces pak choy, trimmed
   strips
Coriander sprigs for
   decoration

Paint duck breasts with 1 tablespoon oil, then rub with Chinese Five-Spice. Heat 1 tablespoon oil in a non-stick pan and cook duck skin side down first until crisp and golden—about 4 minutes. Turn over and cook the other side the same. Turn back to skin up. Place in a pre-heated oven at 400°F for 10 minutes or until cooked to preference, drizzling honey for the last 5 minutes. Heat remaining oil in the duck pan; fry ginger, garlic, and spring onions. Add to duck in roasting pan. Meanwhile, cook pak choy in salted boiling water until just tender. Drain. Spoon ginger and garlic mix onto four warmed serving plates and perch duck breasts on top. Serve with pak choy and decorate with coriander springs. Serves 4.

(*Source:* Courtesy The Honey Association.)

Asian Honey-Tea Grilled Prawns

❖ ❖ ❖

1 cup brewed double strength orange spice tea, cooled
¼ cup honey
¼ cup rice vinegar
1½ pounds medium shrimp, peeled and deveined
¼ cup soy sauce

1 tablespoon fresh ginger, peeled and finely chopped
½ teaspoon ground black pepper
Salt
2 green onions, thinly sliced

In plastic bag, combine marinade ingredients (everything but the shrimp, salt, and onions). Remove ½ cup marinade; set aside for dipping sauce. Add shrimp to marinade in bag, turning to coat. Close bag securely and marinate in refrigerator 30 minutes or up to 12 hours. Remove shrimp from marinade; discard marinade. Thread shrimp onto 8 skewers, dividing evenly. Grill over medium coals 4 to 6 minutes or until shrimp turn pink and are just firm to the touch, turning once. Season with salt, as desired. Meanwhile, prepare dipping sauce by placing reserved ½ cup marinade in small saucepan. Bring to boil over medium-high heat. Boil 3 to 5 minutes or until slightly reduced. Stir in green onions. Serves 4.

(*Source:* National Honey Board.)

Buckwheat Honey Roasted Chicken Breasts with Black Truffle Oil, Yukon Gold Hash, and Grilled Asparagus

❖ ❖ ❖

½ cup olive oil
4 (6 to 8 ounces) airline chicken breasts
Kosher salt
Ground black pepper
½ cup buckwheat honey
4 teaspoons black truffle oil
1½ cups chicken stock
1 tablespoon cold, unsalted butter

½ pound yellow onion, diced small
8 ounces red bell pepper, diced small
2 pounds Yukon gold potatoes, skin on, medium diced
2 tablespoons buckwheat honey
8 ounces green asparagus, peeled

Preheat oven to 300°F, and preheat your grill. In a heavy-bottomed, oven-proof sauté pan, heat 2 tablespoons olive oil. Season the chicken breasts well with salt and pepper. Place the chicken in pan, skin side down. Sear the chicken breasts until the skin is brown and crispy. Turn the chicken breasts over so crispy skin is up. Drain excess oil out of pan. Drizzle approximately ¼ cup buckwheat honey over each chicken breast. Place in preheated oven until cooked through, when a thermometer inserted into the center reaches 165°F, approximately 10 minutes. Drizzle each chicken breast with approximately ½ teaspoon black truffle oil. Remove chicken from pan and set aside. Add chicken stock and stir. Remove cooked-on bits from bottom of pan. Place on stovetop. Bring to a boil, and then reduce to a simmer. Simmer until liquid is reduced by half. Season with salt and pepper. *Monte au buerre* with 1 tablespoon cold, unsalted butter. In a separate, heavy-bottomed sauté pan, heat 4 tablespoons olive oil. Add the onion, peppers, and potatoes. Season well, with salt and pepper. Sauté until all sides of the potatoes are brown and the potatoes are tender, stirring when needed. Prepare asparagus by breaking the stalks where they break naturally. Using a vegetable peeler, peel the bottom one to two inches of the asparagus. Toss well with 2 tablespoons olive oil and season well with salt and pepper. Sear on a hot grill until tender. Slice chicken on a bias, leaving one bone in one piece. Serve with 4 ounces of potato hash, 4 to 6 sprigs of asparagus, and 1 to 2 ounces of sauce. Drizzle each piece of the chicken with approximately ½ teaspoon truffle oil and 1 tablespoon buckwheat honey. Makes 4 servings.

(*Source:* National Honey Board, Orlando Culinary Contest Winner.)

Grilled Honey-Glazed Pork Tenderloin with Onions

❖ ❖ ❖

½ cup buckwheat honey
¼ cup extra virgin olive oil
¼ cup cider vinegar
1 tablespoon minced garlic
2 teaspoons Herbes De Provence seasoning mixture

1 teaspoon salt
½ teaspoon pepper
2 pounds pork tenderloin
2 medium onions

Combine honey, oil, vinegar, garlic, herbs, salt, and pepper in a shallow pan. Add pork and turn to coat well. Cover and refrigerate 2 to 4 hours. Turn pork occasionally. Remove pan from refrigerator 30 minutes before grilling. Prepare grill for medium-hot fire with an indirect heat area. Slice onions in rounds ½- to ¾-inch thick. Remove pork from marinade; turn every 10 minutes to evenly cook. Put onions over direct heat and brush with marinade. Turn frequently brushing with marinade until well marked and soft, 8 to 12 minutes. Move onions off direct heat to finish cooking. Let pork rest 5 minutes before slicing into ¾-inch slices. Serve with grilled onions.

(*Source:* National Honey Board.)

Honey-Glazed Game Hen

❖ ❖ ❖

¼ cup honey
2 tablespoons soy sauce
2 tablespoons lemon juice
½ teaspoon dry mustard
½ teaspoon ground ginger
1 (½ to 1¾ lb.) game hen, thawed
¼ teaspoon salt
⅛ teaspoon pepper
½ onion, peeled and quartered

Combine honey, soy sauce, lemon juice, dry mustard, and ginger in 1-cup microwave-safe measure or bowl; mix well. Microwave at high for 1 to 1½ minutes or until heated; stir to dissolve honey. Rinse game hen and pat dry. Sprinkle cavity with salt and pepper. Dip onion in honey mixture and place 2 quarters in game hen. Tie legs together with heavy string. Place game hen, breast side down, in microwave-safe roasting dish. Brush generously with honey mixture. Microwave at high for 16 to 20 minutes or until juices run clean and meat near bone is no longer pink; rotate rack one-quarter turn every 5 minutes. Turn hen breast side up halfway through cooking time and glaze with remaining sauce. Remove onion from cavity and cut game hen in half. If desired, heat drippings and onion 1½ to 2 minutes in microwave-safe measure; strain and serve with game hen.

(*Source:* National Honey Board.)

Honey Mustard Chicken Tenders

❖ ❖ ❖

1/4 cup Sciabica's or Marsala
Olive Oil or Lavender
Olive Oil
16 chicken tenders
1 egg, slightly beaten
1/3 cup honey
1 tablespoon Dijon mustard

Grated peel of 1 orange or
lemon
1/2 cup fresh basil, chopped
Salt, pepper, and cayenne to
taste
1 tablespoon lemon juice
2 to 3 tablespoons farina or
bread crumbs

In large skillet add olive oil. In mixing bowl add chicken tenders and remaining ingredients except farina. Coat tenders well. Place farina in pie plate. Coat tenders on both sides with farina. Cook on medium heat in olive oil until golden brown, to 170°F. Serve with pasta, potatoes, salad or whatever desired. Serves 4.

(*Source:* Courtesy Gemma Sanita Sciabica, *Cooking with California Olive Oil: Recipes from the Heart for the Heart.*)

Honey Roast Lamb with Couscous

❖ ❖ ❖

2 neck fillets of lamb
1 teaspoon turmeric
1 teaspoon cinnamon
4 tablespoons clear honey
9 ounces couscous
2 onions, sliced

1 garlic clove, crushed
Juice and rind of a lemon
2 ounces pistachio nuts
Small bunch coriander, freshly
　　chopped
Salt and freshly ground black
　　pepper

Preheat the oven to 425°F. Remove any fat from the neck fillets, place in a roasting tin, brush with a little oil, then sprinkle the turmeric and cinnamon. Roast for 10 minutes, then brush with honey and continue to cook for a further 5–10 minutes, depending upon how "well done" you like your meat.

Meanwhile, place the couscous in a bowl and pour over 12 ounces water. Leave to soak for 15 minutes, then steam over a large pan of water in a fine sieve for 35 minutes. When the lamb is cooked, remove from the pan and cover with foil to keep warm. Transfer the cooking juices to a saucepan and add the onions and garlic. Cook over a high heat until the onions are browned and softened.

Stir in the remaining ingredients and then the couscous. Mix through, then transfer to a serving dish. Slice the warm lamb and place over the couscous. Pour over any meat juice, then serve immediately with plenty of freshly chopped coriander. This recipe is also delicious with pork fillet or chicken breast.

(*Source:* Courtesy The Honey Association.)

Marinated Mackerel

❖ ❖ ❖

2 tablespoons clear honey
2 tablespoons wine vinegar
2 tablespoons mil mustard
Salt and freshly ground black
pepper

4 large mackerel, cleaned,
bones removed
4 bay leaves

Mix the honey with the vinegar, mustard, and plenty of seasoning. Lay the fish in a shallow dish and top with bay leaves. Pour over the marinade, cover with cling film, and refrigerate. Leave the fish to marinate for several hours or overnight. Cook the fish opened out under a hot grill, basting frequently with the marinade until it is cooked through. Turn the fish once during cooking. Serve immediately.

(*Source:* Courtesy The Honey Association.)

Pomegranate Glazed Chicken

❖ ❖ ❖

*1 cup 100 percent pome-
    granate juice*
*²/₃ cup Sherry Balsamic
    Vinegar*
¼ cup honey
3 tablespoons brown sugar

4 sprigs fresh thyme
Salt and pepper to taste
*1 whole chicken, skin on, cut
    into pieces (innards
    removed)*
Toasted sesame seeds

Preheat oven to 375°F. In a mixing bowl, combine pomegranate juice, balsamic vinegar, honey, brown sugar, thyme, salt, and pepper. Stir until honey and sugar dissolves. Place chicken pieces in a large Ziploc bag. Carefully pour marinade over them, press air out of bag, and seal. Move bag around to ensure marinade disperses.

Refrigerate bag for 30 minutes. Remove chicken from bag and place in a large glass baking dish, spacing chicken evenly. Bake for 25 to 30 minutes, until chicken is tender but fully cooked. While chicken cooks, carefully pour remaining marinade from bag into a small saucepan over high heat. Bring to a boil (to kill bacteria), then lower heat to medium low and simmer for 12 to 15 minutes until marinade is thick and syrupy. Remove from heat and carefully fish out thyme stems. Once chicken has finished baking, brush glaze over each piece. Sprinkle generously with toasted sesame seeds and serve. Serves 4.

(*Source:* Courtesy The Olive Press.)

Spicy Honey-Pepper Glazed Snapper

❖ ❖ ❖

1 Scotch Bonnet pepper;
  minced
½ tablespoon olive oil
½ cup fresh orange juice
¼ cup plus 1 tablespoon
  Savannah Bee Company
  Grill Honey

1 pinch salt
2 fresh fish: medium / large
  fillets of firm white fish
  like snapper, bass,
  or grouper
Fresh cilantro or basil

FOR THE FISH GLAZE

In a small saucepan sauté the hot pepper in a little olive oil over medium heat. Add the orange juice and bring up to simmer. Simmer for 3 to 4 minutes and then add the honey, stirring quickly to incorporate. Simmer another minute or two until the glaze has a light syrup consistency. Add a pinch of salt.

FOR THE FISH

Prepare your grill and preheat to 375°F. Using tongs, wipe the grill bars with a cloth doused with vegetable oil to clean, and allow 2 minutes to return to full heat. This will score your fillets beautifully. Cook for 5 to 15 minutes per side, depending on fillet thickness, and check doneness as needed. Pour the prepared glaze over the cooked fish before serving. Garnish with fresh cilantro or basil. Serve with steamed bok choy and grilled sweet potato planks.

(*Source:* Courtesy: Savannah Bee Company.)

Spring Rolls

❖ ❖ ❖

3 tablespoons oyster sauce
3 tablespoons light soy sauce
2 tablespoons clear honey
2 cloves garlic, crushed
8 ounces cooked prawns
2 tablespoons oil
Large bunch spring onions,
    chopped

2 tablespoons smooth peanut
    butter
8 ounces fresh bean sprouts
8 ten-inch square sheets frozen
    spring roll pastry, thawed
Oil for deep frying

Mix oyster sauce, soy sauce, honey, and garlic together. Stir in prawns and marinate for about 30 minutes. Lift out prawns and reserve juices. Heat oil in a wok or large frying pan and cook prawns and spring onions for 2 minutes. Stir in reserved juices and peanut butter and cook until sauce begins to thicken. Remove from heat and stir in bean sprouts. Allow to cool. Divide filling between spring roll pastry squares. Fold over one corner and shape the filling into a roll. Fold in the two sides, then roll up lightly. Brush the end with water and slick down. Heat oil and fry two or three at a time, for about three minutes. Keep warm while cooking remainder. Makes 8. For a completely vegetarian dish, omit prawns and replace with a can of drained bean shoots. Makes 8.

(*Source:* Courtesy The Honey Association.)

Desserts

In my younger worker bee days, an older man cooked dinner for me. The salmon was a meltdown because of a rich commercial sauce. Heartburn hit. The salad wasn't fit for a honey bee. Iceberg lettuce is not fit for an iguana. The light-colored greens don't have nutrients like baby spinach with its antioxidants. But the dessert was created for a queen bee. I was served a huge slice of store-bought pound cake, not enough strawberries, gigantic scoops of vanilla ice cream, and whipped cream. I transcended to old-fashioned strawberry shortcake heaven.

These days, I make shortcake with a more sophisticated spin for health nuts who are watching calories, fat, sodium, and cholesterol. First I use a heart-healthy baking mix for the shortcake. Instead of sugar I turn to wildflower honey. I use organic 2 percent low-fat milk and earthy spices: cinnamon and nutmeg. I zap the artificial whipped cream and turn to calcium and vitamin A–rich Häagen-Dazs Vanilla Honey Bee ice cream and drizzle honey on top of the masterpiece. I've got a new crush on my strawberry shortcake fit for a queen bee or her beekeeper with a sweet tooth.

In this section you'll notice that I've included plenty of desserts, because I am a dessert lover. I chose recipes that include common foods of the Oldways Mediterranean Diet and Pyramid. Naturally, *Apple Honey Pie* (an all-American favorite with a taste of honey) is part of the lineup, but other gems include *Baklava, Filo Pear and Honey Tarts, Honey Bee Brownies,* and *Walnut Cake and Honey Lemon Syrup.* Once you begin baking with honey, there's no going back.

Apple Honey Pie
Apricot Honey Crème Bars
Baklava
Butternut Squash and Orange Crème
Carrot, Honey, and Raisin Cake
Chocolate Honey Brûlées
Coconut Custard Pie
Coconut Macaroons
Cranberry Honey Almond Tart
Filo Pear and Honey Tarts
Honey Bee Brownies
Honey Berries with Lime Pound Cake
Honey Oatmeal Cookies
Honey Sesame and Date Biscotti
Struffoli alla Napoletana
Sweet Potato Pie
Walnut Cake and Honey Lemon Syrup

Apple Honey Pie

❖ ❖ ❖

2 cups peeled sliced apples
1 nine-inch pie shell
4 eggs
1 cup plain yogurt

1 teaspoon ground cinnamon
¼ teaspoon salt
¾ cup Sue Bee Honey®
Chopped walnuts

Spread apple slices over pie shell.

Combine eggs, yogurt, cinnamon, salt, and honey to make a custard mixture.

Pour the custard mixture over the apples.

Sprinkle with walnuts.

Bake 45 minutes at 375°F.

Cool to room temperature before cutting. Serves 8.

(*Source:* Courtesy Sue Bee Honey®)

Apricot Honey Crème Bars

❖ ❖ ❖

CRUST
1 cup all-purpose flour
¼ cup sugar
¼ teaspoon salt

½ cup unsalted butter, chilled
   and cut into small bits

FILLING

8 ounces cream cheese,
   softened
1/4 cup sugar
1 large egg, beaten
1 tablespoon lemon juice

1/2 teaspoon pure vanilla
   extract
1/2 cup Honey Ridge Farms
   Apricot Honey Crème
3/4 cup chopped dried apricots

TOPPING

1/2 cup all-purpose flour
1/2 teaspoon baking powder
1/4 teaspoon salt
1/4 teaspoon ground cinnamon
1 cup old-fashioned rolled oats

1/2 cup dark brown sugar
6 tablespoons unsalted butter,
   chilled and cut into small
   bits

TO PREPARE THE CRUST

Preheat the oven to 350°F. Grease a 9x9x2-inch baking pan. In the bowl of a food processor, combine the flour, sugar, and salt and pulse to combine. Add cold butter and pulse until the mixture is crumbly. Pat into the bottom of the prepared pan. Bake about 20 minutes, or until lightly browned.

TO PREPARE THE FILLING

In the bowl of an electric mixer, beat the cream cheese with the sugar. Add the egg and beat until incorporated. Add lemon juice, vanilla, and Apricot Honey Crème and mix well. Stir in the apricots. Pour filling over the crust and spread evenly.

TO PREPARE THE TOPPING

In the bowl of a food processor, combine the flour, baking powder, salt, cinnamon, and brown sugar. Pulse to mix well. Add the chilled butter and pulse until mixture is crumbly. Add the rolled oats and pulse to incorporate. Gently spoon the topping over the filling and pat down gently. Bake about 25 minutes, until bars are golden. Cool, then refrigerate before cutting and serving. Makes 20 servings.

(*Source:* Courtesy Honey Ridge Farms.)

Baklava

❖ ❖ ❖

2 sticks butter
4 cups walnuts (finely chopped)

1 cup sugar
1½ teaspoons cinnamon
1 pound package of phyllo

SYRUP
¼ cup honey
1¼ cups sugar
1¼ cups water
1 lemon rind (cut in chunks) (or a few squeezes of ReaLemon juice)

1 cinnamon stick
4 or 5 whole cloves

Melt butter. Mix chopped nuts, sugar, and cinnamon. Brush a 13" x 9" x 2" glass baking dish with melted butter; sprinkle bottom with cinnamon. Place 3–4 sheets of phyllo on bottom of pan (trim or fold corners as necessary), brush with melted butter, and sprinkle nut mixture on top. Repeat process using only 2 sheets of phyllo per layer, finish with a layer of phyllo only, and brush once more with butter.

Cut halfway through the dessert at a diagonal in either direction to form diamonds. Bake at 300°F for 15 minutes, then 325° for 60 minutes, or until golden brown.

While Baklava is baking, combine all ingredients for the syrup in a heavy-bottomed saucepan (to prevent burning), keep a careful eye on mixture, and stir frequently. Boil for 10 minutes; remove rinds and cloves and let cool for 10 minutes.

(*Source:* Courtesy Bee-Pure Honey®)

Butternut Squash and Orange Crème

❖ ❖ ❖

1 small butternut squash
(about 2 ½ pounds)
1 tablespoon canola oil
1 cup diced silken tofu
¼ cup honey
½ cup fresh orange juice

½ cup commercial vanilla-
flavored soy milk
2 tablespoons grated orange zest
½ cup blueberries, raspberries
or seasonal fruit
⅛ tablespoon grated nutmeg

Preheat the oven to 350°F. Brush the squash with the canola oil; bake for 1 hour and 20 minutes, or until fork-tender. Let cool.

Cut the squash in half. Remove the seeds and discard or save for another use. Scoop out 1 cup of the flesh and transfer it to a blender or food processor fitted with a metal blade. Add the silken tofu, honey, orange juice, soy milk, and orange zest; process until smooth.

Spoon equal portions of berries or other fruit into chilled wineglasses or dessert cups. Pour the crème over the fruit and grate a little nutmeg over the top. Chill for 30 minutes. Serve chilled. Makes 6 servings.

(*Source:* Reprinted with permission from *The Golden Door Spa Cooks Light & Easy* by Chef Michel Stroot, published by Gibbs Smith, 2003.)

Carrot, Honey, and Raisin Cake

❖ ❖ ❖

3 carrots
4 ounces whole meal
   self-raising flour
4 ounces self-raising flour
1 teaspoon baking powder
1 teaspoon cinnamon
1 ounce brown sugar

5 ounces honey
3 eggs
1 teaspoon vanilla extract
4 fluid ounces sunflower oil
3 ounces raisins
2 to 3 tablespoons milk

Preheat the oven to 325°F. Line an 8-inch-round cake tin with grease-proof paper and brush with a little oil. Peel and grate the carrots on a chopping board. Place the flours, baking powder, cinnamon, and sugar in a bowl and mix together. Put the honey, eggs, vanilla, and oil in a separate bowl and mix together with a whisk or fork. Add to the flour mixture and mix well. Stir in the grated carrots and raisins with a metal spoon. Add a little milk to give a fairly soft consistency. Spoon the cake mixture into the lined tin. Bake for about 1 hour. Check that the cake is done by inserting a skewer or knife into it. Leave the cake to cool in the tin for 10 minutes, then loosen the sides and turn out onto a wire rack. Remove the lining paper and leave to cool.

(*Source:* Courtesy The Honey Association.)

Chocolate Honey Brûlées

❖ ❖ ❖

1 can (12 oz.) evaporated milk   *1 tablespoon cocoa powder*
1 cup whole milk   *2 teaspoons grated orange peel*
2 eggs   *1 teaspoon vanilla*
½ cup honey   *3 tablespoons sugar*

In a medium bowl, whisk together evaporated milk, milk, and eggs until well-blended. Mix in honey, cocoa powder, orange peel, and vanilla. Divide mixture evenly between 4 (¾ to 1 cup capacity) oven-proof custard cups or ramekins. Place custard cups in a baking pan. Fill pan with boiling water to reach halfway up cups. Bake at 325ºF 1 hour, or until knife inserted in center comes out clean. Remove cups from baking pan and allow to cool. Cover and refrigerate custard cups until chilled, 4 hours or overnight. Before serving, sprinkle sugar evenly over tops of custards. Place cups under broiler; cook until sugar melts and caramelizes. Makes 4 servings.

(*Source:* National Honey Board.)

Coconut Custard Pie

❖ ❖ ❖

Sure, this type of pie contains sugar and saturated fat, but it's also got protein, calcium, and other minerals, as well as being lower in calories than other pies, such as creamed varieties. If savored in moderation, a small slice isn't a bad thing. Sweets eaten sparingly are included in the traditional Mediterranean diet (it includes eggs) and are not off-limits to the French. Coconut boasts a delightful taste and chewy texture and a bit of dietary fiber and zero cholesterol.

1 store-bought piecrust
⅔ cup granulated sugar
⅓–½ cup organic whole milk or 2 percent organic low-fat milk)
2 tablespoons whole-wheat flour
2 tablespoons European-style butter, cubed
2 large brown eggs, beaten
2 teaspoons orange blossom honey

1 teaspoon orange blossom honey
1 teaspoon pure vanilla extract
Nutmeg
1 cup (plus ⅛ to ¼ cup for topping) shredded coconut, premium brand
Whipped cream
Fresh fruit, such as bananas, peaches, or berries

Preheat oven to 400°F. Take out frozen pie shell and bake for 10 minutes. (This keeps the crust from being soggy when you bake it with the wet ingredients.) Remove from oven and pour in mixture of all ingredients except nutmeg and coconut for topping, the whipped cream, and the fruit. Sprinkle top with nutmeg and coconut (⅛ to ¼ cup, extra). Bake for about 40 minutes at 350° till filling is firm and piecrust is golden. Cool. Slice and garnish with a small dollop of whipped cream and fresh fruit. Serves 8 to 10.

Coconut Macaroons

❖　❖　❖

1/3 cup water
1 cup evaporated cane
  juice
2 tablespoons honey
1/4 teaspoon sea salt

3/4 teaspoon pure vanilla
  extract
1 large egg white
4 cups unsweetened coconut
  flakes

Preheat oven to 350°F. Lightly coat a nonstick baking sheet with canola oil. In a small saucepan, combine water, evaporated cane juice, honey, salt, and vanilla. Bring to a boil. Stir until syrup forms, about 30 seconds. Remove from heat. Combine egg white and coconut flakes in a large bowl. Mix well. Add syrup and mix to form dough. Place 1 tablespoon dough (or use a 1/2-ounce scoop) about 1 inch apart on baking sheet. Bake for 8 minutes. Turn pan and bake for another 4 to 5 minutes, or until light brown. Makes 38 macaroons.

(*Source:* Canyon Ranch.)

Cranberry Honey Almond Tart

❖　❖　❖

1 cup all-purpose flour
1/4 cup granulated white
  sugar
1/4 teaspoon ground cinnamon
1/8 teaspoon salt

1/2 cup cold unsalted butter,
  cut into 1/2-ich cubes
1 large egg yolk, chilled
2 tablespoons heavy cream,
  chilled

In a bowl, whisk together the flour, sugar, cinnamon and salt. Using a pastry blender or two knives, cut in butter until mixture resembles coarse meal. (Or pulse in a food processor fitted with steel blade.)

Mix the yolk with the cream. Add the mixture in the flour mixture, stirring briskly with fork just until moist crumbs forms. Transfer the dough into a 9-inch round tart pan with removable bottom; with floured fingers and dry-measuring cup, press evenly into bottom and up side of pan. Shape and press the edge of dough firmly against side of pan, pushing down with opposite thumb to level top of crust flush with rim. Refrigerate until firm, for at least 30 minutes.

Preheat oven to 425°F. Prick bottom of dough all over with a fork. Line with parchment paper or foil leaving at least a 1-inch overhang. Fill with pie weights or dried beans. Bake for 10 minutes. Turn the heat down to 350°F, bake for 10 minutes. Remove the pie weights and parchment paper. Continue baking until the edges of the crust are just beginning to turn golden and the center looks dry, about 25 to 30 minutes; press with the back of the spoon if it puffs up. Transfer pie shell to a wire rack; let it cool slightly.

FILLING

3 tablespoons unsalted butter

1 cup Honey Ridge Farms Cranberry Honey Crème

4 large eggs

1 teaspoon pure vanilla extract

½ cup toasted sliced almonds

Powdered sugar, for dusting

Preheat the oven to 350ºF. In saucepan, melt the butter over low heat. Remove from heat and add the honey; mix well with a whisk. Add the eggs one at a time, whisking well after each addition. Add vanilla and mix until well combined. Spread half of the almonds on the crust. Pour into the tart shell and bake until center is set, for about 40 to 45 minutes. Remove from pan.

Let it cool completely. Sprinkle with the remaining almonds and dust with powdered sugar. Makes one 9-inch tart or eight 3 ½-inch tarts.

(*Source:* Courtesy Honey Ridge Farms, *Desserts* magazine.)

Filo Pear and Honey Tarts

❖ ❖ ❖

4 conference pears, peeled,
   cored and cut into slices
4 tablespoons clear honey
1 strip orange peel
1 strip of lemon peel
Juice of one lemon

3 tablespoons water
4 sheets of filo pastry
   (approximately 30 cm x 30 cm)
2 tablespoons melted butter
Icing sugar for dusting

Preheat the oven to 350°F. Place the pears, honey, the orange and lemon peel, lemon juice, and water in a large pan and bring to a boil. Lower the heat, cover with a lid, and cook gently for 5 to 7 minutes, stirring occasionally, until the pears are soft. Allow to cool.

Lay the sheets of filo pastry on the work surface and brush lightly with butter. Cut into 16 x 15 cm squares and place another square over the top at an angle to make a star shape. Repeat with 2 more squares of pastry. Gently press into a muffin tin. Repeat with the remaining pastry until you have 4 pastry cases. Fill each case with the pear mixture, then brush the trimmings with butter, scrunch them up, and place on top of the tarts. Bake for 20 to 25 minutes, until golden brown. Serve each tart dusted with icing sugar.

(*Source:* Courtesy The Honey Association.)

Honey Bee Brownies

❖ ❖ ❖

10 ounces unsweetened
  chocolate
6 eggs
3 cups (2 pounds 4 ounces)
  honey

¼ cup vanilla extract
3 cups (14 ounces) biscuit mix
2¾ cups (12 ounces) pecans,
  chopped

Melt chocolate; cool slightly. Beat eggs; beat in chocolate, honey, and vanilla. Thoroughly beat in biscuit mix. Stir in pecans. Pour into greased 12"x20"x2" baking pan; bake at 350°F until toothpick inserted in center comes out clean, about 20 minutes. Cool completely. Spread with Honey Chocolate Frosting, if desired; let set up. Cut into 48 (2"x2½") pieces.

HONEY CHOCOLATE FROSTING

½ cup boiling water
1½ pounds powered sugar
5 ounces unsweetened
  chocolate, melted

¼ cup (3 ounces) honey
½ tablespoon vanilla extract

Gradually beat boiling water into powdered sugar. Beat in melted chocolate, honey and vanilla. Thin frosting with 1–2 tablespoons of boiling water, if necessary. Makes 48 servings.

(*Source:* National Honey Board.)

Honey Berries with Lime Pound Cake

❖ ❖ ❖

LIME POUND CAKE

Canola oil, to coat pan
½ cup unsalted butter
¼ cup low-fat cream cheese
1½ cups evaporated cane juice
3 egg yolks
2¼ cups all-purpose flour
2½ teaspoons baking powder

½ teaspoon baking soda
½ teaspoon sea salt
1 cup buttermilk
¼ teaspoon lime oil
2 tablespoons grated lime peel
3 tablespoons fresh lime juice

HONEY BERRIES

1 cup honey
2½ cups fresh raspberries
2½ cups fresh blackberries

2½ cups fresh blueberries
⅔ cup chopped fresh tarragon

Preheat oven to 350°F. Lightly coat a 9-inch Bundt pan with canola oil. Dust with all-purpose flour.

In a large mixing bowl, cream butter, cream cheese, and evaporated cane juice with an electric mixer on low speed until evaporated cane juice is dissolved and mixture is fluffy. Add egg yolks and mix until combined.

In a medium bowl, sift together flour, baking powder, baking soda, and salt. In another bowl, combine buttermilk, lime oil, lime peel, and lime juice.

Add half of the flour mixture and mix for 30 seconds. Add remaining buttermilk mixture and mix briefly until smooth. Pour batter into Bundt pan. Bake for 40 to 45 minutes, or until toothpick inserted in center comes out clean. Remove from oven and let sit for 15 minutes on a wire rack to cool. Invert cake onto a large plate and let cool completely.

In a medium saucepan, over medium heat, bring honey to a boil. Add berries and toss until well combined. Remove from heat and stir in tarragon. Serve each slice of Lime Pound Cake topped with 3 tablespoons of Honey Berries. Slice into 20 servings.

(*Source:* Canyon Ranch.)

Honey Oatmeal Cookies

❖ ❖ ❖

3 tablespoons butter
½ cup brown sugar
¼ cup Savannah Bee Orange Blossom Honey
1 egg

1 tablespoon water
½ cup flour
½ teaspoon salt
¼ teaspoon baking soda
1 cup rolled oats

Preheat oven to 350°F. Using a mixer with the paddle attachment, mix together thoroughly the butter, brown sugar, honey, egg, and water. Sift together the dry ingredients [except for oats], then stir in the oats. Add the dry ingredients to the wet; mix. Add any additional ingredients like chopped dates, figs, raisins, currents, chocolate chips, chopped nuts—in any amount you like. Drop by heaping teaspoons onto a greased cookie sheet. Bake 12 to 15 minutes. Cool on a wire rack.

(*Source:* Courtesy Savannah Bee Company.)

Honey Sesame and Date Biscotti

❖ ❖ ❖

1½ cups flour
1½ cups whole wheat pastry
    flour
1 teaspoon baking soda
1 teaspoon baking powder
1½ teaspoons five spice powder
⅓ cup Marsala Olive Oil
⅔ cup honey
Grated peel and juice of 1
    small orange

3 eggs
¾ cup dates, dried figs, apricots,
    or fruit of choice
½ cup pecans or nuts of your
    choice, chopped
1 teaspoon vanilla or flavor-
    ing of your choice
¼ cup sesame seeds

Heat oven to 350°F. Lightly grease foil-lined large baking sheet. In mixing bowl combine dry ingredients; make well in center. Pour in olive oil, honey, juice and eggs. Stir until dough holds together; add remaining ingredients (except sesame seeds). Shape dough on lightly floured surface into 4 or 5 logs, 2 by 10 inches long. Place on prepared baking pan, 2 inches apart. Brush tops with milk or water, sprinkle evenly with sesame seeds. Bake 15 to 20 minutes or until firm when lightly touched on top and golden. Remove to cutting board; cool. Cut logs into about ½ inch slices, diagonally. Place back on baking sheet, cut side down. Bake 4 to 5 minutes to toast until golden brown. Makes 60 to 70.

(*Source:* Courtesy Gemma Sanita Sciabica, *Baking with California Olive Oil: Dolci and Biscotti Recipes.*)

Struffoli alla Napoletana

❖ ❖ ❖

1¾ cups flour
½ teaspoon salt
1 teaspoon baking powder
¼ cup sugar
Grated peel of 1 orange or 1
  lemon

3 small eggs
1 teaspoon vanilla
4 tablespoons Marsala Olive Oil
  for cooking struffoli (2 or 3
  inches in small saucepan

SYRUP
⅓ cup honey
⅓ cup water

¼ cup sugar

DECORATIONS
¼ cup candied red and green
  cherries, chopped small
¼ cup candied orange or
  pumpkin, diced

½ cup pine nuts or walnuts,
  chopped
⅓ cup dark chocolate, chopped
  small

In mixing bowl combine dry ingredients; make well in center. Add eggs, vanilla, and olive oil; stir until dough holds together. Knead very little, on floured board; cover; let rest about 30 minutes. On lightly floured board, pinch off small pieces of dough. Roll to thickness of a pencil (about ¼ inch). Cut each roll into ½-inch pieces; roll to form little balls. Cook a few at a time in heated olive oil until golden brown. Remove with a slotted spoon onto pan lined with clean paper towels. In a small saucepan bring to boil honey, water, and sugar. Stir to dissolve; simmer 1 minute. Remove from heat; cool. Dip struffoli into syrup with candied ingredients, pine nuts, and chocolate. Place in a pile or pyramid on a plate. Serves 6.

Note

Struffoli may be baked on lightly greased cookie sheets. Place little balls on sheets with a little space in between each one. Bake in a 350-degree oven for 15 to 20 minutes or until golden brown.

(*Source:* Courtesy Gemma Sanita Sciabica, *Baking with California Olive Oil: Dolci and Biscotti Recipes.*)

Sweet Potato Pie

❖ ❖ ❖

7 cups cooked and mashed
  sweet potatoes
1/4 teaspoon ground nutmeg
1 teaspoon ground cinnamon
2 tablespoons vanilla extract
2 teaspoons lemon juice

2 1/4 cups sugar
1 cup Savannah Bee
  Company Orange
  Blossom Honey
4 jumbo eggs
2 deep-dish pie shells

Preheat oven to 350°F. Place sweet potatoes, nutmeg, cinnamon, vanilla, lemon juice, sugar, Savannah Bee Company Orange Blossom Honey, and eggs in a large bowl. Blend ingredients together until they are thoroughly mixed. Equally distribute the sweet potato mix into the pie shells. Place some aluminum foil on and around the edges of the pie shells so the crust will not burn when the pies are baked. Place pies in the oven and bake for 45 minutes. Remove from the oven and let cool completely before serving. Serve with whipped cream. Makes 2 pies / 16 to 20 servings.

(*Source:* Courtesy Savannah Bee Company.)

Walnut Cake and Honey Lemon Syrup

❖ ❖ ❖

6 eggs, separated
1½ cups walnuts, ground
1¾ cup flour
½ teaspoon soda
1 teaspoon cinnamon
¼ teaspoon ginger or cloves
1 cup sugar
1½ teaspoons baking powder

½ teaspoon salt
¼ teaspoon nutmeg
Grated peel of 1 lemon or
   tangerine
¾ cup yogurt, plain
¼ cup Marsala Olive Oil
1 teaspoon orange extract

HONEY LEMON SYRUP
½ cup sugar
⅓ cup honey
Juice of 2 lemons

Peel of 1 lemon, grated
⅓ cup water

Preheat oven to 350°F. Grease a 13 x 9 inch baking pan. In mixing bowl, add egg whites. Beat until stiff peaks hold. In another bowl, add dry ingredients. Make well in center. Add yogurt, olive oil, orange extract, and egg yolks; stir to blend well. Gently fold in egg whites; pour into prepared pan. Bake for 30 to 40 minutes, or until center springs back when touched lightly on top in center. Cool on wire rack. In saucepan combine sugar, honey, lemon juice, lemon peel, and water. Bring to a boil. Lower heat, simmer two minutes, cool. Poke holes all over top of cake with tines of fork. Spoon syrup over top of cake, if desired. Makes 16 pieces.

(*Source:* Courtesy Gemma Sanita Sciabica, *Baking Sensational Sweets with California Olive Oil.*)

A Final Buzz

*The sweetest honey
Is loathsome in his own deliciousness
And in the taste confounds the
appetite.*

—William Shakespeare[1]

These days, as a citified mountain woman—a nature girl at heart—I sit here amid towering pine trees and inside a human hive full of honeys from the honey bee and its people. My pantry is stuffed full with honey varietals that I know intimately and continue to use in cooking, baking, and of course tea, as well as straight from the spoon. Candles, all types, tapers to pillars, are in every room; the kitchen, dining room, living room, bedroom, study, and bathroom.

I am inspired by the honey varietals around the world and the variety of healing powers that are linked to each one. I confess that I do like the milder, lighter varieties, such as wildflower and orange blossom, but leatherwood and buckwheat intrigue me and my palate. The benefits of beeswax, from the incredible beauty products to soaps, have pampered my body and spirit in the comfort of my cabin.

SELF-RELIANCE AND THE QUEEN BEE MENTALITY

Still, today in the 21st century there are doctors, nutritionists, and everyday people, maybe even you, who believe honey is just a sweetener that's good on toast or in tea. Honey is so much more than that. Take 1 teaspoon of honey for energy and please go back to chapter 1. Reread my words, chapter by chapter, to get the message that honey has amazing healing powers, thanks to the gifted honey bee. Here are four tips I follow day to day.

Queen Bee Tip 1: Listen to your body's cues. I've tuned into my vital signs, whether it be monitoring my blood pressure or aches and pains that zap energy. This way, you'll be on top of any problem and can nip it in the bud—and honey can help.

Queen Bee Tip 2: Eat premium, whole natural foods (think royal jelly and the queen) to help you treat your body like royalty. It's about taking care of yourself, first and foremost, so you can be productive in your hive— and honey can help.

Queen Bee Tip 3: Stay busy. Being productive and knowing what your purpose in life is will help you feel focused and keep you heart-healthy and your weight in check—and honey can help.

Queen Bee Tip 4: Stay in touch with your health-care practitioner: Make sure you have a caring doctor, much like an attentive beekeeper, who can help you keep tabs on your overall health with preventative care. It will give you peace of mind so you can do what you want to do in life—and honey can help.

So, as I come to an end of sharing Honeyland with you, it's no surprise that I feel connected to the honey bee. Through human years I have transformed from a traveling human like a virgin queen to a queen bee comfortable in her hive to produce products, like *The Healing Powers of Honey*, to help mankind bee healthy. And it's honey (and bee foods straight from the hive) that has and will continue to make my life sweeter (and yours, too) through middle age and into the golden years. Like a queen I am happy to say, "Honey, I'm home."

PART 9

HONEY
RESOURCES

Where Can You
Buy Honey?

As honey continues to be touted for its powerful health benefits, people are becoming more aware of this ancient superfood and its comeback around the globe. Currently, a wide world of honeys can be bought in supermarkets, specialty stores, and health-food stores, as well as through mail order and on the Internet. And yes, the decision regarding which one is best can be subjective, just like when choosing your favorite olive oil and chocolate.

Here is a list of honeys and honey products, from organic and all-natural to gourmet brands. If you're interested in buying any of these popular honeys or honey-related items, just contact the honey company directly for the locations of stores nearest you.

HONEY BEAUTY PRODUCTS

Bella Luccè
Bella Luccè Ltd. Co.
401 Western Lane
Suite G
Columbia, S.C. 29063
800-485-3079
Outside the lower 48 states:
803-749-0809
www.bellalucce.com

Manuka Honey Drizzle, one of the company's most popular products, can be used as a pedicure soak, as a hydrotherapy bath treatment, and as a rich body masque.

Cuccio Naturalé
29120 Avenue Paine
Valencia, CA 91355
661-257-7827; 800-762-6245
www.cuccio.com

In 1999, the innovative Star Nail International founded
the first natural nail-, hand-, and foot-care treatment
product line used in top spas and salons worldwide. Many
of the products, from massage crèmes to Spa Elixir, include milk-and-honey combinations and are simply sublime—perfect for pampering the body at home, too.

HONEY HOUSEHOLD PRODUCTS

Big Dipper Wax Works
700 South Orchard Street
Seattle, WA 98108
206-767-7322; 888-826-7770
www.bigdipperwaxworks.com

Hand-crafted beeswax candles. Products include tapers, pillars, and gift sets for everyday and extraordinary seasonal selections: holiday glass gift sets, Scents of the Season, beehive glasses, Valentine's Day candles, and a spring collection.

Honey Candle
37 Main Street
Orleans, MA 02653
508-255-7031; 888-423-3929
www.honeycandle.com

Quaint candle shop, 100 percent beeswax collection, pillars, tapers, bayberry candles, and summer butterflies on front and back of decorative candles.

Knorr Beeswax Products, Inc.
14906 Via De La Valle
Del Mar, CA 92014
760-431-2007; 800-807-BEES
www.knorrbeeswax.com

Beeswax candles are pure elegance and perfect for all occasions. Selection of quality 100 percent pure beeswax candles.

HONEY PRODUCERS AND MAKERS IN CALIFORNIA

Honey Pacifica
www.honeypacifica.com

Honey Pacifica offers raw honey varieties, always raw and unfiltered. A wide variety of exceptional honeys, honeycomb, candy, coastal bee pollen, royal jelly, propolis, skin creams and lip balms, and beeswax candles.

Honey Ridge Farms
12310 NE 245th Avenue
Brush Prairie, WA 98606
360-256-0086
www.honeyridgefarms.com

Unforgettable gourmet honey, honey crèmes, honey vinegar, and honey grilling sauces and glazes.

Marshall's Honey
159 Lombard Road
American Canyon, CA 94503
707-556-8088; 800-624-4637
www.marshallshoney.com

California honey, raw honey, kosher honey, unfiltered honey, allergy relief packs, and beeswax products.

HONEY COMPANIES FROM OTHER STATES IN THE USA AND AROUND THE GLOBE

Banner Bee Company LLC
10021 Banner County
Laytonsville, MD 20882
240-793-0363
www.bannerbees.com

An eye-catching selection of quality honey products, including raw honey, beeswax candles, gourmet cocoa blended raw honey, and all-natural HelpingHand propolis salve.

Bee-Pure Honey, Inc.
West Bend, WI 53095
262-675-0557
www.beepurehoney.com

Provides natural, healthy honey and other hive products, including bee pollen, gift sets, raw honey, and tea, direct from the beekeeper.

Laney Honey
25725 New Road
North Liberty, IN 46554
574-656-8701
www.laneyhoney.com

Premium honey from America's Heartland, varieties offered by floral source, as well as beeswax and skin-care products.

Dutchman's Gold
300 Carlisle Road
Carlisle, ON
LOR 1H2, Canada
905-689-6371
www.beepollenbuzz.com
www.dutchmansgold.com
www.anniesapitherapy.com

Raw, fresh, and unpasteurized honey varietals and honey blends, including fresh comb honey, raw honey, summer blossom honey, honey butter, and buckwheat honey. Apitherapy raw honey blends, including royal jelly, bee propolis, and bee pollen for added nutritional value.

Magnolia Honey Company
Post Office Box 517 / 251 Highway 61 North
Woodville, MS 39669
601-888-7500
www.magnoliahoney.com

Home of award-winning gourmet products, including honey jellies, honey pickles, and honey sauces.

Really Raw Honey
3725 Gough Street
Baltimore, MD 21224
800-REAL-RAW (732-5729)
www.reallyrawhoney.com

An earthy line of a variety of raw honeys, including unprocessed honey containing bits of propolis, honeycomb, and pollen that add chewy texture.

Savannah Bee Company
211 Johnny Mercer Boulevard
Savannah, GA 31410
800-955-5080
www.savannahbee.com

A top-notch company with a vast assortment of specialty honeys, raw honeycomb, everyday honey, body-care products, and gifts.

Sue Bee® Honey
301 Lewis Boulevard
P.O. Box 338
Sioux City, IA 51102
712-258-0638
www.suebee.com

A leading honey company in America, which offers all-natural honey, spun honey, Aunt Sue's Raw Honey with pure unfiltered all natural flavor, and Aunt Sue's Organic Honey, which is certified 100 percent organic as recognized by the USDA.

Volcano Island Honey Company, LLC
46-4013 Puaono Road
Honokaa, HI 96727
808-775-1000; 888-663-6639
www.volcanoislandhoney.com

Raw honey fit for the gods. Tropical honey is certified organic.

GOURMET SPECIALTY FOODS

ChefShop.com
1425 Elliott Avenue West
Seattle, WA 98119
800-596-0885
www.ChefShop.com

ChefShop.com carries an extensive line of artisan-produced specialty foods and ingredients from around the world, including a broad selection of monofloral honeys, such as Tasmanian leatherwood honey and Tasmanian tea tree honey. Stop by the retail store anytime to try honey or ask for a personalized olive oil and vinegar tasting. Or shop online.

MEDICINAL HONEY

During the creation of *The Healing Powers of Honey,* as an author-intuitive I was working as a phone psychic. I'd get calls from Australia and New Zealand. Often, I'd sense the caller (sometimes without an accent) was ringing me from these countries. It was just a gut instinct.

Honeymark International, LLC
P.O. Box 15381
Boston, MA 02215
866-427-7329
www.HoneymarkProducts.com

A wide variety of imported medicinal honey products, including first-aid antiseptic lotion, antifungal cream, liquid hand soap, and manuka honey soap. The manuka honey is the only product imported from New Zealand. These soaps are excellent for moisturizing dry skin, clearing acne, and eliminating bacteria on the surface of the skin.

Medihoney
Derma Sciences
214 Carnegie Center
Suite 300
Princeton, NJ 08540
609-514-4744
www.medihoney.com

Linked to Comvita, Medihoney was a pioneer in the field of honey and wound-care research.

The Tasmanian Honey Company
25A Main Road
Perth, Tasmania 7300
Australia
(03) 6398 2666
www.tasmanianhoney@microtech.com.au

A potpourri of delicious and sophisticated honeys with healing properties, including Tasmanian leatherwood, Tasmanian manuka, French lavender, and eucalyptus.

Comvita New Zealand Ltd
Private Bag 1, Te Puke
New Zealand
0800-504-959
www.comvita.com

A pioneer company selling honey and other bee products, including manuka honey, first-aid creams, and honey bandages.

The Honey Collection Limited
74 Grove Road
Blenheim 7201
Marlborough
New Zealand
+64-3-5786303
www.honeycollection.co.nz

The Honey Collection provides a variety of "Pure New Zealand Skin Care products" that have UMF-rated manuka honey as a prime ingredient.

CHOCOLATE TO PAIR WITH HONEY

Lake Champlain Chocolates
750 Pine Street
Burlington, VT 05401
800-465-5909
www.lakechamplainchocolates.com

For 25 years, Lake Champlain Chocolates has been making fresh, all-natural gourmet chocolates.

Natural Candy Store
1009 Shary Circle, Suite B
Concord, CA 94518
925-288-1704; 800-875-2409
www.naturalcandystore.com

Honey candies, including Italian Honey Filled Candy, Honey Mint Patties, Honeybees Natural Candy, and much more.

Queen Bee Gardens
1863 Lane 11 1/2
Lovell, WY 82431
307-548-2543; 800-225-7553
www.queenbeegardens.com

A wide variety of the best gourmet candy made with honey and chocolate, including truffles, Honeymoons, pralines, and other confections.

OLIVE OIL TO PAIR WITH HONEY

Nick Sciabica & Sons
2150 Yosemite Boulevard
Modesto, CA 95354-3931
209-577-5067; 800-551-9612
www.sciabica.com

Sciabica specializes in cold-pressed olive oils, using several varieties of California olives. They also provide natural red wine vinegar, as well as balsamic vinegar imported from Modena, Italy. Sciabica offers a variety of extra virgin olive oils. Also, Sciabica's "Specialty Olive Oils" include flavored products containing basil, garlic, jalapeño, lemon, and orange. These oils contain no artificial flavors but are made by crushing and cold-pressing together the ingredients and fresh Mission Variety olives in the mill.

The Olive Press
At Jacuzzi Family Winery
24724 Highway 121 (Arnold Drive)
Sonoma, CA 95476
707-939-8900; 800-965-4839
www.theolivepress.com

The Olive Press Tasting Room and Gift Shop and the online store are dedicated to olives and olive oil. They also sell some honey-related items, including Olive You Dog Treats that come in peanut butter and honey.

Tea to Pair with Honey

Celestial Seasonings
The Hain Celestial Group, Inc.
4600 Sleepytime Drive
Boulder, CO 80301
800-434-4246
www.celestialseasonings.com

All-natural chai, green, herbal, red, wellness, white, and specialty teas with honey are what you'll find at Celestial Seasonings, the largest specialty tea manufacturer in North America. Honey teas include Honey Vanilla Chamomile Herbal Tea, Sweet Apple Chamomile Herbal Tea, Honey Lemon Ginseng Green Tea, and Honey Vanilla Chai Tea.

BUZZ-WORTHY INFORMATION ON HONEY

Bee Culture
623 W. Liberty Street
Medina, OH 44256
330-725-6677; 800-289-7668
www.BeeCulture.com

Bee Culture was established in 1873 and has been published by the A. I. Root Company, in Medina, Ohio, since its inception. Readers are international but mostly from the U.S. and reflect the beekeeping community... about 10 percent commercial, 25 percent sideliners, and the rest backyard beekeepers.

Canadian Honey Council—National Office
36 High Vale Crescent
Sherwood Park, AB
Canada
T8A 5J7
877-356-8935; 780-570-5930
www.honeycouncil.ca

Committee for the Promotion of Honey and Health, Inc.
P.O. Box 3
Haddam, KS 66944-0003
713-436-7802
www.prohoneyandhealth.com

The Honey Association
Grayling Portland House
Bressenden Place
London,
SW1E 5BH
+44-0-20-7932-1850
www.honeyassociation.com

UK honey site, compiled by British Honey Importers and Packers Association. Contains honey recipes and honey health tips.

The Honey Locator
11409 Business Park Circle
Suite 210
Firestone, CO 80504
303-776-2337
www.honeylocator.com

The Honey Locator is a valuable resource that dishes out suppliers of honeys and products in the United States. You can pinpoint an apiary state by state, or you can search by honey type.

National Honey Board
11409 Business Park Circle
Suite 210
Firestone, CO 80504
303-776-2337
www.honey.com

The National Honey Board was founded in 1990 to enlighten the public about all things honey related, from the honey bee and honey health benefits to honey facts and recipes. Its goal is to educate people about honey use by consumers, the food industry, and food manufacturers.

Notes

CHAPTER 1:
THE POWER OF HONEY

1. "Honey Quotes," www.foodreference.com/html/qhoney.html.
2. Steven G. Pratt, M.D., and Kathy Matthews, *SuperFoods HealthStyle: Simple Changes to Get the Most Out of Life for the Rest of Your Life* (New York: Harper, 2007), p. 148.
3. Jonny Bowden, Ph.D., C.N.S., *The 150 Healthiest Foods on Earth: The Surprising, Unbiased Truth About What You Should Eat and Why* (Beverly, MA: Fair Winds Press, 2007), p. 316.

CHAPTER 2:
AN ANCIENT ESSENTIAL ELIXIR

1. "Famous Honey Quotes," www.honeything.com/articles/honey quotes.html.
2. Nathanial Altman, *The Honey Prescription: The Amazing Power of Honey as Medicine* (Rochester, VT: Healing Arts Press, 2010).
3. Ibid, page 45.
4. Ibid, page 44.
5. Jenni Fleetwood, *Honey: Nature's Wonder Ingredient:*

100 Amazing Uses from Traditional Cures to Food and Beauty, with Tips, Hints, and 40 Tempting Recipes (London: Lorenz Books, 2007), page 12.

6. Ibid, page 14.

7. Ibid, page 14, 15.

8. Jenni Fleetwood, *Honey: Nature's Wonder Ingredient: 100 Amazing Uses from Traditional Cures to Food and Beauty, with Tips, Hints, and 40 Tempting Recipes* (London: Lorenz Books, 2007), p. 15.

9. Nathanial Altman, *The Honey Prescription: The Amazing Power of Honey as Medicine*, p. 56.

10. Jenni Fleetwood, *Honey: Nature's Wonder Ingredient: 100 Amazing Uses from Traditional Cures to Food and Beauty, with Tips, Hints, and 40 Tempting Recipes* (London: Lorenz Books, 2007), p.15.

11. The National Honey Board; http://www.honey.com/nhb/media/press-kiet/press-kit-honey-history-facts/.

12. Jenni Fleetwood, *Honey: Nature's Wonder Ingredient: 100 Amazing Uses from Traditional Cures to Food and Beauty, with Tips, Hints, and 40 Tempting Recipes* (London: Lorenz Books, 2007).

13. Ron Fessenden, MD, MPh.H, and Mike McInnes, MRPS, *The Honey Revolution: Restoring the Health of Future Generations* (Haddam, KS: World Class Emprise, LLC, 2008), p. 142.

CHAPTER 3:
A HISTORICAL TESTIMONY

1. "Bee Quotes." www.brainquote.com/quotes/keywords/bees.html.

2. Douglas Martin, "Eva Crane, English Expert on World's Bees, Dies at 95," the *New York Times*, Sep-

tember 16, 2007, www.ny times.com/2007/09/16/world/europe/16crane.html.

3. Peter Marren, "Eva Crane: Authority on the History of Beekeeping and Honey-Hunting Who Traveled the World in Pursuit of Bees," *The Independent*, September 14, 2007, www.independent.co.uk.

4. "Global Honey Market to Reach 1.9 Million Tons by 2015, According to New Report by Global Industry Analysts, Inc.," San Jose, California (PRWEB), February 8, 2010: www.prweb.com/releases/honey_honeybee/raw_monoflorz/_polyfloral/prweb3453 434.htm.

CHAPTER 4:
WHERE ARE THE SECRET INGREDIENTS?

1. "Honey Quotes," www.foodreference.com/html/qhoney/html.

2. Steven G. Pratt, M.D., and Kathy Matthews, *SuperFoods HealthStyle: Simple Changes to Get the Most Out of Life for the Rest of Your Life* (New York: Harper, 2007), p. 147.

3. Nele Gheldof, Xiao-Hong Wang, and Nicki J. Engeseth, "Buckwheat Honey Increases Serum Antioxidant Capacity in Humans," *J. Agric. Food Chem.* 51 (5) (February 26, 2003): 1500–1505.

CHAPTER 5:
HONEY, YOU'RE AMAZING!

1. "Famous Honey Quotes," www.honeything.com/articles/honey quotes.html.

2. Jonny Bowden, Ph.D., C.N.S., *The 150 Healthiest Foods on Earth: The Surprising, Unbiased Truth About*

What You Should Eat and Why (Beverly, MA: Fair Winds Press, 2007), p. 223.

3. Allen R. Robin, et al., "Daily Consumption of a Dark Chocolate Containing Flavanols and Added Sterol Esters Affects Cardiovascular Risk Factors in a Normotensive Population with Elevated Cholesterol," *American Society for Nutrition J. Nutr.* 138 (April 2008): 725–731.

4. "Malaysian Honey Retards Cancer Growth, Inhibits Bacteria and Fungi," *Apitherapy News,* February 9, 2010, www.apitherapy.blogspot.com.2010/02/maylasian-honey-retards-cancer-growth.html.

5. "Buzz Surrounds Venom in Cancer Research," The Day, retrieved August 5, 2010 www.theday.com/article/2010805/B1202/308059461/1/B12.

6. Mike and Stuart McInnes, *The Hibernation Diet* (Haddam, KS: World Class Emprise, LLC, 2007), p. 7.

7. Ron Fessenden, MD, MPH, and Mike McInnes, MRPS, *The Honey Revolution: Restoring the Health of Future Generations* (Haddam, KS: World Class Emprise, LLC, 2008), p. 125.

8. H. Guo, A. Saiga, et al., *J. Nutr. Sci. Vitaminol.* (Tokyo) 53 (4) (August 2007): 345–348. R&D Center, Nippon Meat Packers, Inc.

9. Ray Sahelian, MD, "Royal Jelly Benefit, Side Effects, Research Information of this Health Supplement," www.raysahelian.com/royaljelly.html.

10. C. R. Earnest, et al, "Effects of Preexercise Carbohydrate Feedings on Glucose and Insulin Responses During and Following Resistance Exercise," *Strength and Conditioning Research* 14 (2000) 361.

11. www.comvita.com/aboutus/html.

12. "Honey as an Aphrodisiac," www.hubpages.com/hub/Honey_as_ an_Aphrodisiac, by Princessa.

CHAPTER 6:
THE MEDITERRANEAN SWEETENER

1. "Honey Quotes," www.foodreference.com/html/qhoney.html.
2. "New Antioxidant Compounds Have Been Identified in Foods Such as Olive Oil, Honey and Nuts Using Two Analytical Techniques," November 20, 2009, www.medicalnewstoday.com/articles/171618.php.
3. Daphne Miller, M.D., *The Jungle Effect: A Doctor Discovers the Healthiest Diets from Around the World—Why They Work and How to Bring Them Home* (New York: HarperCollins, 2008), p. 54.

CHAPTER 7:
HEALING HONEY VARIETIES

1. "Honey Quotes," www.foodreference.com/html/qhoney.html.
2. Bob Gulliford, "Beginning in Bees," *The Australian Beekeeper,* August 2010, p. 83.
3. Ibid., p. 83.
4. Jenni Fleetwood, *Honey: Nature's Wonder Ingredient: 200 Amazing Uses from Traditional Cures to Food and Beauty, with Tips, Hints and 30 Tempting Recipes* (London: Lorenz Books, 2008), p. 30.

CHAPTER 8:
HONEY AND CINNAMON POWER

1. www.quotesea.com/quotes/keywords/cinnamon.
2. Steven G. Pratt, M.D., and Kathy Matthews, *SuperFoods HealthStyle: Simple Changes to Get the Most Out of*

Life for the Rest of Your Life (New York: Harper, 2007), pages 281–282.

3. Ibid., p. 282.

CHAPTER 9:
SWEET STUFF: HONEY COMBOS

1. "Honey Quotes," www.foodreference.com/html/qhoney/html.

2. "Global Honey Market to Reach 1.9 Million Tons by 2015, According to New Report by Global Industry Analysts, Inc.," San Jose, California (PRWEB), February 8, 2010.

CHAPTER 10:
TEA(S) WITH YOUR HONEY

1. "Tea and Toast Food Quotes," www.foodreference.com/html/qteaandtoast.html.

CHAPTER 11:
HOME REMEDIES FROM YOUR KITCHEN

1. "Famous Honey Quotes," www.honeything.com/articles/honeyquotes .html.

2. D. C. Jarvis, M.D., *Folk Medicine: A New England Almanac of Natural Health Care from a Noted Vermont Country Doctor* (New York: Fawcet Crest Books, 1958), p. 115.

3. Ibid., pp. 115–116.

4. Ibid., p. 109.

5. Ibid., p. 112.

6. E. A. Ophori, B. N. Eriagbonyer, and P. Vgbodaga,

"Antimicrobial Activity of Propolis Against *Streptococcus mutans*," *African Journal of Biotechnology* 9 (31) (August 2, 2010): 4966–4969.

7. I. M. Paul, J. Beiler, A. McMonagle, et al., "Effect of Honey, Dextromethorphan, and No Treatment on Nocturnal Cough and Sleep Quality for Coughing Children and Their Parents," *Arch. Pediatr. Adolesc. Med.* (12) (December 2007): 1140–1146.

8. Jarvis, *Folk Medicine*, p. 109.

9. Douglas I. Rosendale, et al., "High-through Put Microbial Bioassays to Screen Potential New Zealand Functional Food Ingredients Intended to Manage the Growth of Probiotic and Pathogenic Gut Bacteria," *International Journal of Food Science & Technology* 43 (12) (November 2008): 2257–2267.

10. Howland Blackiston, *Beekeeping for Dummies* (Hoboken, NJ: Wiley Publishing, 2009), p. 31.

11. Cal Orey, *The Healing Powers of Vinegar* (New York: Kensington Books, 2009), p. 175.

12. Ibid, p. 214.

13. Jarvis, *Folk Medicine*, p. 119.

14. Ibid.

CHAPTER 12:
HONEYMANIA: HONEY FOR THE HOUSEHOLD

1. "Famous Honey Quotes," www.honeything.com/articles/honeyquotes.html.

2. "Did You Know You Can Use Honey to Treat a Wound on Your Pet?" *K9 Magazine,* May 1, 2009, www.dogmagazine.net/archives.

CHAPTER 13:
HONEY BEE-AUTIFUL

1. "Famous Honey Quotes," www.honeything.com/articles/honeyquotes .html.
2. "Prince Charles' Wife Uses Bee Venom, Honey to Fight Wrinkles: Camilla Fights Wrinkles with 'Bee Venom.'" *PTI*, July 28, 2010.

CHAPTER 14:
THE BUSY BEE WORKERS

1. "Famous Honey Quotes," www.honeything.com/articles/honeyquotes .html.

CHAPTER 15:
HONEY IS NOT A BUZZ FOR EVERYONE: THE STING

1. www.quotesdaddy.com/quote/934659/Joseph_Jouber/when-you-go-in-search-of-honey-you-must-expect-to.
2. Tom Keyser, "Bee Venom Used to Treat Arthritis, MS, Lupus, Chronic Fatigue Syndrome," *Times Union*, February 1, 2009.
3. Ray Sahelian, MD, "Royal Jelly Benefit, Side Effects, Research Information of this Health Supplement," www.raysahelian.com/royaljelly.html.
4. Andrew Schneider, Senior Public Health Correspondent, "11 Execs, 6 Foreign Firms Caught in Honey Sting," September 2, 2010, www.aol news.com.
5. Ray Sahelian, MD, "Honey Health Benefit," www.ray sahelian.com/honey.html.

6. Charles Downey, "Sweet Solution," WebMD, March 13, 2000: www.medicinenet.com/script/main/art.asp?articlekey=50608.

CHAPTER 16:
AND THE BEES' BUZZ GOES ON . . .

1. Oscar Wild, from "Her Voice," *Poems 1881*.
2. Allison Aubrey, "Healing Honey and the New Queen Bee-(keepers)" July 19, 2010, www.npr.org/2010/07/19/128574280/healing-honey-and-the-new-queen-bee-keepers.

CHAPTER 17:
THE JOY OF COOKING WITH HONEY

1. "Honey Quotes," www.foodreference.com/html/qhoney.html.

CHAPTER 18:
CIAO, HONEY!

1. "Honey Quotes," www.thinkexist.com/quotes/ with keyword/ honey.
2. "All About Honey," February 29, 2000, www.virtual-weberbullit. com/honey.html.
3. "Honey Quotes," www.foodreference.com/html/qhoney.html.

Selected Bibliography

Altman, Nathaniel. *The Honey Prescription: The Amazing Power of Honey as Medicine.* Rochester, VT: Healing Arts Press, 2010.

Blackiston, Howland. *Beekeeping for Dummies.* Hoboken, NJ: Wiley Publishing, 2009.

Bowden, Jonny, Ph.D., C.N.S. *The 150 Healthiest Foods on Earth: The Surprising, Unbiased Truth About What You Should Eat and Why.* Beverly, MA: Fair Winds Press, 2007.

Fessenden, Ron, MD, MPH, and Mike McInnes, MRPS. *The Honey Revolution: Restoring the Health of Future Generations.* Haddam, KS: World Class Emprise, LLC, 2008.

Fleetwood, Jenni. *Honey: Nature's Wonder Ingredient: 200 Amazing Uses from Traditional Cures to Food and Beauty, with Tips, Hints and 30 Tempting Recipes.* London: Lorenz Books, 2008.

Jarvis, D. C., M.D. *Folk Medicine: A New England Almanac of Natural Health Care from a Noted Vermont Country Doctor.* New York: Fawcett Crest Books, 1958.

Marchese, Marina C. *Honeybee: Lessons from an Accidental Beekeeper.* New York: Black Dog & Leventhal Publishers, 2009.

McInnes, Mike and Stuart. *The Hibernation Diet.* Haddam, KS: World Class Emprise, LLC, 2007.

Pratt, Steven G. M.D., and Kathy Matthews. *SuperFoods*

HealthStyle: Simple Changes to Get the Most Out of Life for the Rest of Your Life. New York: Harper, 2007.

Sciabica, Gemma Sanita. *Baking Sensational Sweets with California Olive Oil.* Modesto, CA: Gemma Sanita Sciabica, 2005.

————. *Baking with California Olive Oil: Dolci and Biscotti Recipes.* Modesto, CA: Gemma Sanita Sciabica, 2002.

————. *Cooking with California Olive Oil: Popular Recipes.* Modesto, CA: Gemma Sanita Sciabica, 2001.

————. *Cooking with California Olive Oil: Recipes from the Heart for the Heart.* Modesto, CA: Gemma Sanita Sciabica, 2009.

————. *Cooking with California Olive Oil: Treasured Family Recipes.* Modesto, CA: Gemma Sanita Sciabica, 1998.

Traynor, Joe. *Honey: The Gourmet Medicine.* Bakersfield, CA: Kovack Books, 2002.

Connect with Us

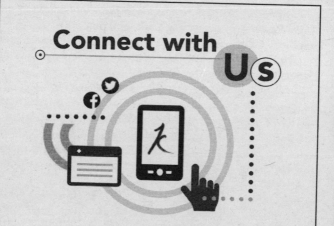

Visit us online at
KensingtonBooks.com
to read more from your favorite authors, see books
by series, view reading group guides, and more.

for sneak peeks, chances to win books and prize packs,
and to share your thoughts with other readers.

facebook.com/kensingtonpublishing
twitter.com/kensingtonbooks

Tell us what you think!

To share your thoughts, submit a review,
or sign up for our eNewsletters, please visit:
KensingtonBooks.com/TellUs.